MRCP PART 2: CASE HISTORIES AND DATA INTERPRETATIONS

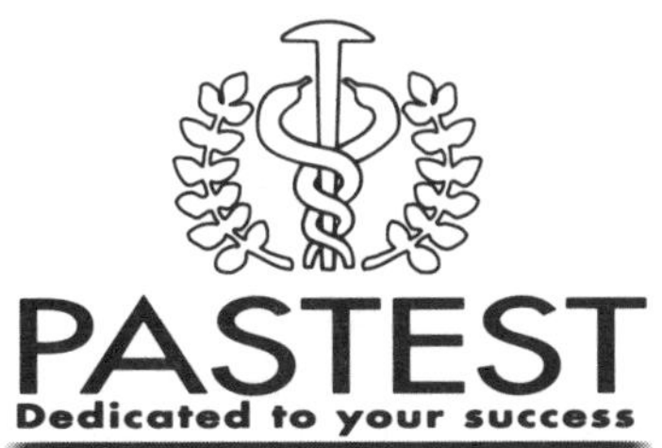

Cover Slides:

- Chest X-ray: Fallot's tetralogy, coeur-en-sabot
- CT: Adult polycystic disease
- Blood film: Myeloma, plasma cells and rouleaux formation courtesy of the Haematology department, Christie Hospital
- ECG: Wolff-Parkinson-White Syndrome type B

MRCP PART 2: CASE HISTORIES AND DATA INTERPRETATIONS

Hans-Ulrich Laasch MD, MRCP, FRCR
Cook Interventional Fellow
Department of Diagnostic Radiology
South Manchester University Hospitals

© 2000 PASTEST
Egerton Court
Parkgate Estate
Knutsford
Cheshire WA16 8DX

Telephone: 01565 752000

First published 2000

ISBN 1 901198 33 2

A catalogue record for this book is available from the British Library.

Typeset by Breeze Ltd, Manchester.
Printed by Bell and Bain Ltd, Glasgow.

CONTENTS

PREFACE

The second part of the MRCP examination has seen some interesting changes in 1999. Firstly, the number of attempts is no longer limited to six. Secondly, a multiple choice type format has been introduced in all three parts of the written exam (Slide, Data and Case History sections). We thought that this would make the questions easier to answer however, this is not so! Minor details in the history often only discriminate between the two best possible answers. It must, however, be remembered that the exam is **not** negatively marked and it is therefore foolish to leave any questions unanswered. Thirdly, a bare fail in the written part (9/20 marks) now only requires one extra mark to be gained in the clinical section, as opposed to the three marks previously required. In theory this should make the exam easier to pass, in practice the vast majority of candidates fail on the short cases. A bare fail in the shorts (5/10) or in the long case (4/8) still requires 3 additional marks from the other three parts, thus increasing the total pass mark to 27. The most important aspect for passing the exam is practice. This applies to the clinical part even more than for the written. First-timers do not usually realise that the 4-6 weeks between the written and clinical part is generally *insufficient time* to practise all the examination routines for heart, chest, abdomen, CNS, cranial nerves, legs... Reading material for the Viva, besides the BMJ editorials, should include Drugs and Therapeutics Bulletin, CMOS-update and the Sunday papers.

It must be remembered that the exam is set so that overall only 25–30% of all candidates pass. The most enthusiastic and knowledgeable teachers for MRCP often had three or four, or even all six attempts at the exam. Although the College is trying to make the exam more objective, a good portion of luck is required on the day. This book is an attempt to repay all the help I have received from my friends and consultants on my way to membership. A special thanks goes to Dr Datta-Chaudhuri and Dr Downton from the Care of the Elderly Department in Stockport. I also need to thank my wife for her patience as well as her continued input into this work. Finally, if there is one piece of advice that summarises my experience:

There is no substitute for having seen or done it before.

Best of luck

HUL

REVISION TIPS FOR THE MRCP PART 2 WRITTEN PAPERS

The written section of the MRCP Part 2 exam consists of three papers with equal marks assigned to each. It is not necessary to achieve a particular mark for each paper as long as the aggregate for all three reaches the required level (10/20). In the written 8 marks equal a clear fail and the candidate will not be allowed to proceed to the clinicals. It is possible to proceed to the clinical exams with a marginal fail in the written (9/20). In this case you will need to make up an extra mark in the clinical to achieve the pass mark, in order to pass overall. Since Autumn 1999 it is no longer required to gain 3 extra marks in the clinical to compensate for a bare fail in the written.

The MRCP Part 2 exam aims to be a test of competent clinical practice, with increasing emphasis on decision-making, as opposed to the theoretical knowledge required for Part 1. There is no doubt that efficient, systematic preparation for the Part 2 can make all the difference between passing and failing the examination.

Approximately 73–75% of candidates pass the written papers but of these only about 30–35% succeed in the clinicals. However, do not wait for the results of the written exam before preparing for the clinical.

Familiarise yourself with the type of questions being asked, how best to present your answers and how they are marked, as this will help you to do justice to yourself in the exam.

Legibility is essential. A weary examiner may not give you the benefit of doubt. If you are desperate you should at least describe what you see. There is no negative marking so you have nothing to lose and may well pick up a mark or two. Multiple Choice Questions (MCQs) and Extended Matching Questions (EMQs) are now a feature of Part 2 and are likely to increase in number in the future. Best-out-of-five questions represent the majority of questions in this book, some old-style questions are included in each chapter as these are still in use by the college.

Failure can be due to lack of knowledge, technique or both:

- Give some thought to how you are going to structure your learning and revision. This includes your time at work, at home and when on courses.
- When revising questions write down your answers, as written

evidence of your decision. This will commit you to your answers and will get you into the habit of writing out your answers in their most complete form.

- Do practice questions under exam conditions i.e. give yourself a strict time limit.
- Give as much information as possible in your answers. Answers are ranked according to quality. When answering a question fullness and precision is required (i.e. complete left side oculomotor nerve palsy with pupillary sparing).
- If asked for three answers, don't give four. The fourth will be ignored.
- Look at the written exam as a way of optimising your chance of passing the whole exam. Aim at a mark of 12–13 rather than just a pass. It will provide a cushion for the clinical exam.

CASE HISTORIES

There are three types of question:

1. **The standard grey case** as seen in many books e.g. give three causes/three useful investigations etc.
2. **The extended answer question.** The information is provided followed by relevant questions then further information etc. The information may include pictures or data allowing the question to be built up into a complete case.
3. **The one-best-answer question**. Here the questions are finely balanced questions depicting several potential answers as a variation on the theme. This type of question is becoming more popular as it tests decision-making rather than simple planning of management of investigation. This requires less writing but more thought!

The questions related to the four or more cases are designed to test your diagnostic skills and your ability to plan further appropriate investigations and outline a management plan. Some questions will provide you with a series of possible answers which will test your ability to decide upon the best course of management.

This paper is difficult to prepare for but many questions do conform to recognised patterns. Thus it is important that you employ a logical technique to approaching each case. Some cases are straightforward. Some cases are truly grey. Practice as many questions as possible.

- Highlight or underline the hard facts in the history and the results. Remember that some items of information will be essential to the differential diagnosis but occasionally some may be 'red herrings'.
- Look carefully at the given history for pointers i.e. age, ethnic origin, profession, unusual symptoms, family history etc.
- Identify abnormalities – usually abnormal laboratory results and physical signs.
- Construct differential diagnoses from the investigations, physical examination and salient features in the history. Then narrow down your differential diagnosis by cross indexing your differentials until you reach the most likely diagnosis.
- Remember that hard facts (i.e. blood results, radiology, ECGs) often show you why one diagnosis is superior to the rest. They can also be crucial to direct you to a diagnosis in a truly grey case. Once you understand the reason for the hard facts ensure the softer points, usually historical, fit the diagnosis.
- When looking at giving answers to confirm diagnosis, remember histology is the usual gold standard.
- Be precise, give as full an answer as possible to gain full marks, but do not write an essay or waffle.
- Do not use abbreviations (e.g. CXR) unless this features in the question as an abbreviation.
- Do not skip over unusual symptoms/signs or other pieces of information as these may give the main clue to the diagnosis.
- If asked for 3 investigations after 3 differential diagnoses, give the best (most diagnostic) investigation possible for each of the differential diagnoses.
- Time yourself carefully. If you are having trouble move on to the next case and come back to it later.

DATA INTERPRETATIONS

The questions related to the 10 sets of data are designed to test not only your understanding of a range of laboratory/radiological investigations and their importance in clinical diagnoses, but also how well you are able to integrate information and to summarise your answers clearly and concisely. This type of question is under review by the college regarding predictability.

Questions include ECGs, echocardiograms, cardiac catheter studies, 'specialised' data (such as family pedigree or audiograms), biochemistry, haematology and pulmonary function tests.

- During your revision take each specialty at a time and try to predict the investigations about which you might be questioned.
- 'Practice makes perfect.' Most questions are variants on a theme which will become apparent if sufficient questions are undertaken.
- You will be expected to know 'normal ranges' for common investigations.
- There are often difficult examples of common investigations and more straightforward examples of specialist investigations.
- Apply common sense and basic principles.
- Practice a logical approach to the data which will help you to arrive at the correct diagnosis i.e. as you would examine the various components of the ECG, one at a time.
- Work through mock papers under exam conditions and time yourself carefully leaving 10 minutes at the end for a recap.
- Again, when attempting a mock paper, don't look at the answers until you have finished and written in your best answers. Always commit yourself to an answer to make the most value of that question.
- Keep strictly to time, miss out questions that you find difficult to come back to later.

PHOTOGRAPHIC MATERIAL

Breadth of knowledge is important as almost anything can be shown. Try to see as many cases as possible.

- Practice logical methods of looking at photographs. Be certain you are familiar with the normal picture, so that you are able to identify subtle abnormalities (tropical medicine, haematology and ophthalmology are difficult, so get enough exposure and practice in these areas).
- Look at as many slides and photos as possible before the exam.
- Have a system for looking at radiographic pictures before the exam. See as many different slides and photos of the same disease process as you can to understand why it is what it is, and that you have not just recognised one particular photo.
- Common investigations are popular, such as blood films and CXR.
- Prepare lists of common conditions likely to be presented.

RETAKING

- If you are retaking try and understand why you failed
- Concentrate on your areas of weakness
- You can significantly improve your exam performance with good technique
- Think about the way you learn, is it as effective as it could be?
- Keep referring to your revision timetable
- Use your daily work to help you learn
- Do you work best by yourself or as part of a group?
- Keep motivated
- Plan your revision so you are at a peak when you take the exam. A weekend course just before the exam can often provide this impetus and motivation.
- Practice, practice, practice on good quality mock exam questions. Be sure to work on the new set of past papers from The Royal College expected Spring 2000.

Good Luck!

PASTEST

CARDIOLOGY QUESTIONS: CASE HISTORIES

For 'best-of-five' questions candidates must select one answer only, by putting a cross in the appropriate box.

Case History 1 (9 marks)

A 59-year-old bachelor is admitted to the A&E Department with acute central abdominal pain. The pain has come on while lifting a crate of beer out of the car and has become worse over the ensuing two hours, it is exacerbated by movement and deep inspiration. Over the last year he has noticed a decline in exercise tolerance, but has put this down to 'old age'. He has developed an irritating nocturnal cough, and a salbutamol inhaler prescribed by the GP has given no relief.

On examination he is pale and sweating and there is guarding and rebound tenderness in the umbilical region. No organomegaly is felt. Pulse rate 124/min, irregular, BP 105/60 mmHg. There is a right parasternal heave and a low frequency diastolic murmur is auscultated over the apex. The chest is clear except for minimal crackles at the lung bases.

Investigations show:

Hb	121 g/l
WCC	11.3 x 10^9/l (83% granulocytes)
Plt	301 x 10^9/l
MCV	79 fl
ESR	41 mm/hr
Na	138 mmol/l
K	5.0 mmol/l
Urea	10.3 mmol/l
Creatinine	156 µmol/l
Chloride	93 mmol/l
Bilirubin	21 U/l
AST	61 U/l
ALT	73 U/l
Arterial blood gases (on air):	
pH	7.31
pO_2	10.9 kPa (82 mmHg)
pCO_2	4.1 kPa (31 mmHg)
Bicarbonate	18 mmol/l
O_2-sat.	97%

Chest X-ray: Mild cardiomegaly, pulmonary congestion, left main bronchus elevated
ECG: Fast atrial fibrillation, 1 mm ST-depression in V_5 and V_6.

1. What is the cardiac abnormality?

- ❑ A Mitral stenosis
- ❑ B Atrial septal defect
- ❑ C Atrial myxoma
- ❑ D Mitral regurgitation
- ❑ E Ruptured chordae tendineae
- ❑ F Dressler syndrome

2. What is the cause for the acute presentation?

- ❑ A Posterior myocardial infarction
- ❑ B Pulmonary embolus
- ❑ C Pericarditis
- ❑ D Hepatitis
- ❑ E Mesenteric infarction

3. What is the cause of the acid-base abnormality?

- ❑ A Acute hepato-cellular injury
- ❑ B Alveolar hypoventilation
- ❑ C Acute renal failure
- ❑ D Lactic acidosis
- ❑ E Aspirin overdose

4. Which of the following investigations is urgently indicated?

- ❑ A Echocardiogram
- ❑ B Mesenteric angiogram
- ❑ C Barium enema
- ❑ D Ventilation-perfusion scan
- ❑ E Serology for atypical infection

Case History 2 (8 marks)

A 24-year-old patient with learning difficulties is referred for investigation of hypertension. He works as a helper in the local garden centre with a particular interest in herbs. There is a family history of hypertension and heart disease.

On examination he is of short stature with under-developed secondary sexual characteristics. He has mild dyspnoea at rest, but is not cyanosed. Pulse 96/min, regular, BP 195/100 mmHg in both arms. The apex beat is thrusting and a loud mid-systolic murmur is heard throughout the precordium radiating into the neck and back. Crackles are audible at both lung bases, examination of the abdomen is unremarkable.

The following results are obtained:

Hb	143 g/l
WCC	5.5 x 10^9/l (normal differential)
Plt	183 x 10^9/l
ESR	8 mm/hr
Na	138 mmol/l
K	4.1 mmol/l
Creatinine	92 µmol/l
Urinalysis	Protein +, Blood -

ECG: QRS-axis -15°, sinus rhythm 98/min, QRS 0.11 sec.
$S_{V2}+R_{V5}$ = 51 mm

A chest X-ray of poor quality could only be obtained as the patient was frightened by the X-ray machine, however cardiomegaly is present and there is dilatation of the ascending aorta.

1. **What is the cardiac diagnosis?**

- ❑ A Hypertrophic obstructive cardiomyopathy
- ❑ B Sub-valvular aortic stenosis
- ❑ C Coarctation
- ❑ D Patent ductus arteriosus
- ❑ E Ventricular septum defect

2. Which of the following is the least useful investigation?

- ☐ A Echocardiogram
- ☐ B MR-scanning
- ☐ C Cardiac szintigraphy
- ☐ D Cardiac catheterization
- ☐ E Angiography

3. What is the likely underlying condition?

- ☐ A Turner's syndrome
- ☐ B Noonan's syndrome
- ☐ C Klinefelter's syndrome
- ☐ D Hurler's syndrome
- ☐ E Homocysteinuria

4. What treatment would you recommend?

- ☐ A Antibiotic prophylaxis
- ☐ B ACE-inhibitors
- ☐ C Calcium-antagonists
- ☐ D Indomethacin
- ☐ E Surgery

Case History 3 (6 marks)

A 54-year-old woman is referred by her GP with a six-month history of shortness of breath, malaise and weight gain. She was successfully treated for lymphoma in her twenties, but this was complicated by tuberculosis at the time. Two years previously she had a severe flu-like illness with pleuritic chest pain which resolved with symptomatic treatment only.

On examination she is overweight but otherwise well. Her jugular venous pressure is raised 6 cm above the sternal angle with systolic collapse. The cardiac apex cannot be palpated, the heart sounds are soft and no murmurs are heard. Pulse 92/min, regular, BP 110/55 mmHg. There is bilateral pitting oedema of the ankles. Examination of the abdomen reveals no abnormality.

Blood results show:

Hb	114 g/l
WCC	4.9 x 10^9/l (normal differential)
Plt	219 x 10^9/l
ESR	21 mm/hr
Na	133 mmol/l
K	5.5 mmol/l
Creatinine	198 μmol/l
Total cholesterol	6.1 mmol/l
LDL	4.3 mmol/l (< 3.9 mmol/l)
Glucose	6.3 mmol/l

Chest X-ray: Large globular heart, lungs clear except for some apical calcification

1. What is the cardiological diagnosis?

- ❑ A Constrictive pericarditis
- ❑ B Myocarditis
- ❑ C Endo-myocardial fibrosis
- ❑ D Pericardial effusion
- ❑ E Restrictive cardiomyopathy

2. Which of the following is the least likely precipitating cause?

- ❑ A Recurrent lymphoma
- ❑ B Gout
- ❑ C Hypothyroidism
- ❑ D Tuberculosis
- ❑ E Bornholm disease

3. What treatment would you recommend?

- ❑ A Digoxin
- ❑ B ACE-inhibitors
- ❑ C Pericardial fenestration
- ❑ D Systemic steroids
- ❑ E Thyroxine

Case History 4 (7 marks)

A 28-year-old man, who was awaiting an appointment in the Cardiology Clinic for repeated syncopes, is admitted as an emergency after collapsing in the gym. On arrival, he is unconscious without cardiac output. His brother indicates that there is a strong family history of cardiac disease, but he is on no current medication.

The monitor shows a broad complex tachycardia of variable amplitude, no pulse is palpable, there is no respiratory effort and the pupils are small.

1. **What is the correct management?**

- ❑ A Precordial thump, DC-shocks, epinephrine 1:1,000 iv
- ❑ B DC-shocks, intubation and cardiac compressions
- ❑ C 1:5 CPR, iv fluids, chest aspiration
- ❑ D DC-shocks, 1:15 CPR, epinephrine 1:10,000 iv
- ❑ E External pacing, adenosine iv, carotid sinus massage

During resuscitation the arrhythmia terminates spontaneously and the patient remains stable.

The following results are obtained:

Na	142 mmol/l
K	5.9 mmol/l
Urea	6.2 mmol/l
Creatinine	141 µmol/l

Arterial blood gases:	
pH	7.28
pO_2	19.7 kPa (148 mmHg)
pCO_2	7.7 kPa (58 mmHg)
Bicarbonate	13 mmol/l
O_2-sat.	100%

ECG: Sinus rhythm 168/min, axis +90°, PQ 0.1 sec. QRS 0.09 sec. Corrected QT 0.50 sec., 1 mm ST elevation in V_4 to V_6

2. What is the likely underlying cause?

- ❑ A Hyperkalaemia
- ❑ B Wolff-Parkinson-White syndrome
- ❑ C Romano-Ward syndrome
- ❑ D Jervell-Lang-Nielsen syndrome
- ❑ E Lown-Ganong-Levine syndrome

3. What was the nature of arrhythmia?

- ❑ A Ventricular tachycardia
- ❑ B Junctional tachycardia
- ❑ C Ventricular fibrillation
- ❑ D Torsade-de-Pointes tachycardia
- ❑ E AV-re-entrant tachycardia

Case History 5 (8 marks)

A 62-year-old man is admitted to Coronary Care with an acute anterior myocardial infarction. He is treated with r-TPA and makes an initially uneventful recovery. One week later he complains of increasing breathlessness and is found to be hypotensive.

On examination the venous pressure is raised and a new systolic murmur is heard through the precordium. Bilateral crackles are present at both bases, pulse 112/min, regular, BP 80/45 mmHg, respiratory rate 28/min.

The ECG shows no new changes, a chest X-ray shows bilateral peri-hilar oedema.

A right-sided cardiac catheter delivers the following measurements for the pulmonary artery:

Pressure	43/14 mmHg
Capillary wedge pressure	10 mmHg
O_2-sat.	91%

1. **What is the likely diagnosis?**
2. **What is your next investigation?**
3. **What management would you recommend?**

Case History 6 (6 marks)

A 21-year-old woman is under investigation for hypertension. She also gives a several month history of malaise and dizzy spells. On examination she looks well, without evidence of anaemia or jaundice. Her right radial pulse is weak, the left radial pulse is absent. Blood pressure measurements give the following results:

Right arm 85/45 mmHg	Left arm unrecordable
Right leg 180/100 mmHg	Left leg 175/105 mmHg

The following blood results are obtained:

Hb	133 g/l
WCC	6.2 x 10^9/l (normal differential)
Plt	343 x 10^9/l
ESR	56 mm/hr
Na	136 mmol/l
K	5.1 mmol/l
Urea	7.9 mmol/l
Creatinine	171 µmol/l
Dipstix urine	Blood ++, Protein -, Glucose -

A carotid Doppler shows occlusion of the right internal carotid artery.

1. What is the likely cause for the hypertension?

- ❑ A Aortic aneurysm
- ❑ B Aortic occlusion
- ❑ C Coarctation
- ❑ D Renal artery stenosis
- ❑ E Chronic renal failure

2. What is the likely diagnosis?

- ❑ A Marfan's syndrome
- ❑ B Takayasu's arteritis
- ❑ C Pseudoxanthoma elasticum
- ❑ D Conn's syndrome
- ❑ E Kawasaki syndrome

Case History 7 (10 marks)

A 56-year-old man is admitted for increasing shortness of breath and confusion. He was well until a week ago when his wife noticed increasing dyspnoea and some erratic behaviour.

In the past he has been investigated for two episodes of haematuria, but iv urography, cystoscopy and ultrasound one month previously had not detected any abnormality. He had hepatitis A at the age of 23 and rheumatic fever and endocarditis as a child.

On examination he is orientated to person but not to time and place. He is hyper-reflexic in left arm and leg, with a slight increase in tone but no other focal signs. Pulse 120/min, irregular, JVP elevated 4 cm, soft pan-systolic murmur at the apex radiating to the axilla. Auscultation of the chest reveals a mild wheeze and bilateral basal crackles. The spleen can be palpated 1 cm below the costal margin, the liver is not enlarged and there is no lymphadenopathy.

The following results are obtained:

Hb	128 g/l
WCC	9.3 x 10^9/l
Plt	476 x 10^9/l
CRP	21 mg/dl (< 10 mg/dl)
Na	139 mmol/l
K	4.6 mmol/l
Urea	10.1 mmol/l
Creatinine	172 μmol/l
Bilirubin	18 U/l
AST	34 U/l
Dipstix urine	Blood ++, Protein +, Glucose -

ECG: Atrial fibrillation, 116/min, QRS axis +15°, 1 mm ST depression in the lateral leads.

1. Which of the following sets of investigations is the most useful?

❑ A White cell differential, chest X-ray, urine culture and microscopy
❑ B ESR, abdominal ultrasound, cardiac enzymes
❑ C Repeat IVU, hepatitis serology, left-sided cardiac catheter
❑ D Echocardiogram, blood cultures, CT brain
❑ E Creatinine clearance, CT kidneys, right-sided cardiac catheter

2. What management would you recommend?

- ❑ A 100% O_2 and oral sotalol
- ❑ B iv antibiotics and iv furosemide
- ❑ C iv fluids and iv digoxin
- ❑ D iv diamorphine and renal dose dopamine
- ❑ E Insertion of central line and iv amiodarone

3. What is the likely diagnosis?

- ❑ A Endocarditis
- ❑ B Renal cell carcinoma
- ❑ C Pyelonephritis
- ❑ D Transitional cell carcinoma
- ❑ E Peri-nephric abscess

4. What complication has arisen?

- ❑ A Cerebral metastasis
- ❑ B Cerebral abscess
- ❑ C Subarachnoid haemorrhage
- ❑ D Subdural empyema
- ❑ E Cerebral haemorrhage

Case History 8 (10 marks)

A tall 19-year-old woman presents to the Casualty Department with an acute episode of severe central chest and back pain. There is a family history of diabetes and ischaemic heart disease. The only past medical history includes a motorbike accident two years previously. She smokes 15 cigarettes per day and her only medication is the oral contraceptive pill.

On examination she looks unwell. Pulse 104/min, regular, BP 105/50 mmHg in the right arm, and 160/65 mmHg in the left arm. The jugular venous pressure is raised 4 cm with a normal wave-form. The right carotid pulse is weak, the left is impalpable. The heart sounds are normal. A short diastolic murmur is audible at the left sternal edge and basal crackles are present at both bases.

Investigations reveal the following results:

Hb	142 g/l
WCC	6.3 x 10^9/l
Plt	229 x 10^9/l
ESR	17 mm/hr
Na	141 mmol/l
K	4.3 mmol/l
Urea	5.2 mmol/l
Creatinine	78 µmol/l

Chest X-ray: Cardio-thoracic ratio 61%, upper mediastinal widening, upper lobe blood diversion
ECG: Sinus rhythm 108/min, QRS axis +60°, 3 mm ST elevation in leads II, III and aVF

1. What is the diagnosis?

- ❑ A Aortic thrombosis
- ❑ B Aortic dissection
- ❑ C Rupture of aortic pseudo-aneurysm
- ❑ D Haemorrhagic pericarditis
- ❑ E Superior vena cava syndrome

2. What complications have arisen? (Tick any that apply)

❑ A Myocardial infarction
❑ B Pericardial effusion
❑ C Aortic incompetence
❑ D Rupture of papillary muscle
❑ E Left sub-clavian artery occlusion
❑ F Left ventricular rupture
❑ G Left common carotid occlusion

3. Which of the following investigations is not indicated?

❑ A Blood cultures
❑ B Contrast-enhanced CT thorax
❑ C Carotid Doppler
❑ D Fundoscopy
❑ E Aortic arch angiogram

4. What underlying cause has to be considered?

❑ A Previous trauma
❑ B Pseudoxanthoma elasticum
❑ C Buerger's disease
❑ D Panarteritis nodosa
❑ E Marfan's syndrome

Case History 9 (5 marks)

A 66-year-old diabetic patient is admitted with a two-day history of pleuritic chest pain and exercise-induced dyspnoea. In the past he had required a triple bypass eight months previously for worsening ischaemic heart disease. He had made an uneventful recovery, now only requiring nitro-glycerine spray two to three times per month. His current medication is enalapril for microalbuminuria and mild hypertension, 75 mg aspirin and intensified insulin therapy. On examination the patient has a temperature of 38.3°C, the chest is clear. The heart sounds are quiet, no murmurs are heard. Pulse 92/min, regular, BP 125/70 mmHg. Sharp anterior central chest pain is provoked by deep inspiration. Examination of the abdomen is normal. Investigations reveal the following results:

Hb	134 g/l
WCC	8.8 x 10^9/l (normal differential)
Plt	398 x 10^9/l
ESR	43 mm/hr
Na	140 mmol/l
K	4.0 mmol/l
Urea	12 mmol/l
Creatinine	153 μmol/l

ECG: Sinus rhythm 90/min, QRS axis 0°, concave ST elevation of 2–3 mm in the anterior chest leads

Chest X-ray: Mild cardiomegaly, moderate pulmonary congestion and small right pleural effusion

1. What is the likely diagnosis?

- ❑ A Silent myocardial infarction
- ❑ B Viral pericarditis
- ❑ C Left ventricular aneurysm
- ❑ D Auto-immune pericarditis
- ❑ E Myocarditis

2. What is the treatment?

- ❑ A Anti-coagulation
- ❑ B Pericardial fenestration
- ❑ C Indomethacin
- ❑ D Steroids
- ❑ E Streptokinase

Case History 10 (7 marks)

A 17-year-old male complains of rapid palpitations associated with dizziness and shortness of breath. The episodes are self-limiting and not clearly related to exercise. There is no previous history of note. On examination he is thin with a malar flush and mild central cyanosis and a raised venous pressure with a prominent systolic wave. Pulse 80/min, regular, BP 115/75 mmHg. A pan-systolic murmur is heard at the left sternal edge, accentuated on inspiration. There is mild, pulsatile hepatomegaly. Examinations reveal:

Full blood count	Normal
Urea & Electrolytes	Normal
ESR	5 mm/hr

ECG: Sinus rhythm 80/min, PR 0.10 sec. A delta wave and an incomplete right bundle branch block pattern are present in keeping with Wolff-Parkinson-White syndrome Type A

1. What is the most important investigation?

❑ A Chest X-ray
❑ B Blood cultures
❑ C Echocardiogram
❑ D Cardiac catheterization
❑ E 24-hour cardiac monitoring

2. What is the likely diagnosis?

❑ A Corrected transposition of the great arteries
❑ B Fallot's tetralogy
❑ C Ostium primum atrial septal defect
❑ D Patent ductus arteriosus
❑ E Ebstein's anomaly

3. What is the likely form of his arrhythmias?

❑ A Sinus tachycardia
❑ B AV re-entrant tachycardia
❑ C Paroxysmal atrial fibrillation
❑ D Intermittent AV-block
❑ E Ventricular tachycardia

Case History 11 (7 marks)

A 43-year-old woman is admitted after having collapsed at home. The preceding weeks she has complained of some tiredness, but has not required any time off work. There is no past history of note.

On examination she is drowsy with weakness of all four limbs. There is no neck stiffness or papilloedema. Auscultation reveals no murmurs, but a loud third heart sound. There is no clinical evidence of cardiac failure. She is admitted and makes a general improvement overnight. However, the nursing staff point out that her eyesight now seems extremely poor. There is no residual weakness, she is alert and orientated and does not complain of any visual disturbances. Fundoscopy, eye movements and pupillary light reflexes are normal. However, she is unable to count fingers.

Examinations reveal:

Hb	139 g/l
WCC	4.6 x 10^9/l (normal differential)
Plt	401 x 10^9/l
ESR	56 mm/hr
Na	142 mmol/l
K	4.8 mmol/l
Creatinine	105 µmol/l
Albumin	40 g/l
Total protein	95 g/l
AST	28 U/l

ECG: Sinus rhythm 64/min, QRS axis +60°, no ischaemic changes
Chest X-ray: Normal heart and lungs

1. **What is the cause for her acute presentation?**
2. **What is the underlying cause?**

Case History 12 (8 marks)

A 15-year-old boy is admitted with headaches, palpitations and nausea. On examination he is pale, has mild photophobia, but is fully alert and orientated. Auscultation of heart and chest reveal no abnormalities. The abdomen is tender, bowel sounds are increased but no mass or organomegaly can be palpated. Pulse 100/min, regular, BP 195/110 mmHg, respiratory rate 18/min.

Preliminary investigations show:

Hb	153 g/l
WCC	4.9 x 10^9/l (normal differential)
Plt	271 x 10^9/l
ESR	8 mm/hr
Na	142 mmol/l
K	3.6 mmol/l
Urea	8.9 mmol/l
Creatinine	109 μmol/l

1. Which of the following is the least likely diagnosis?

- ❑ A Cocaine abuse
- ❑ B Nephroblastoma (Wilms' tumour)
- ❑ C Renal artery stenosis
- ❑ D Conn's syndrome
- ❑ E Amphetamine overdose

The patient is resuscitated and further investigations show the following results:

Liver function tests	Normal
Dipstix urine	Blood -, Protein +, Bilirubin -

ECG: QRS axis -15°, sinus rhythm 92/min, $S_{V2} + R_{V5} = 4.2$ mV, T-inversion V_5 and V_6
Ultrasound abdomen: Normal, liver, spleen and kidneys

2. Which of the following investigations would you recommend?

- ❑ A Renal angiogram
- ❑ B Urinary catecholamines
- ❑ C Chest X-ray
- ❑ D CT abdomen
- ❑ E Urinary 5-(OH) indol-acetic acid

The patient is prepared for surgery.

3. What are two important pre-operative measures?

- ❑ A Estimation of creatinine clearance and octreotide administration
- ❑ B Administration of beta-blockers and bronchodilators
- ❑ C Salt-free diet and aspirin
- ❑ D Administration of ACE-inhibitors and diuretics
- ❑ E iv rehydration and α-blockade

CARDIOLOGY QUESTIONS: DATA INTERPRETATIONS

For 'best-of-five' questions candidates must select one answer only, by putting a cross in the appropriate box.

Data Interpretation 1 (4 marks)

A 56-year-old man is under investigation for atypical chest pains. The following ECG was acquired during an exercise test. The patient has reached Stage II of the standard Bruce protocol.

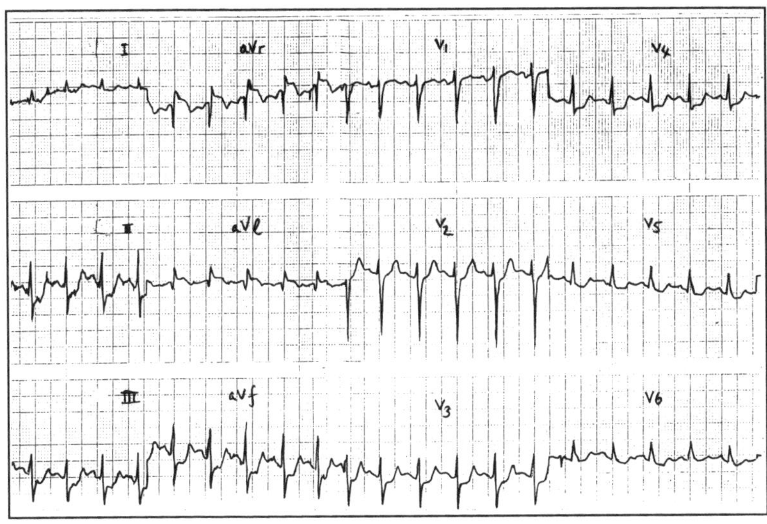

1. How do you interpret the ECG?

- ❑ A Insignificant changes
- ❑ B Significant ischaemia
- ❑ C Acute myocardial infarction
- ❑ D Old myocardial infarction
- ❑ E Left ventricular hypertrophy

2. What further investigation would you recommend?

- ❑ A Echocardiogram
- ❑ B Barium swallow
- ❑ C Thallium myocardial szintigraphy
- ❑ D Gastroscopy
- ❑ E Coronary angiography

Data Interpretation 2 (3 marks)

This is a ST-segment analysis from a 24-hour tape in a man complaining of intermittent central chest pain at rest.

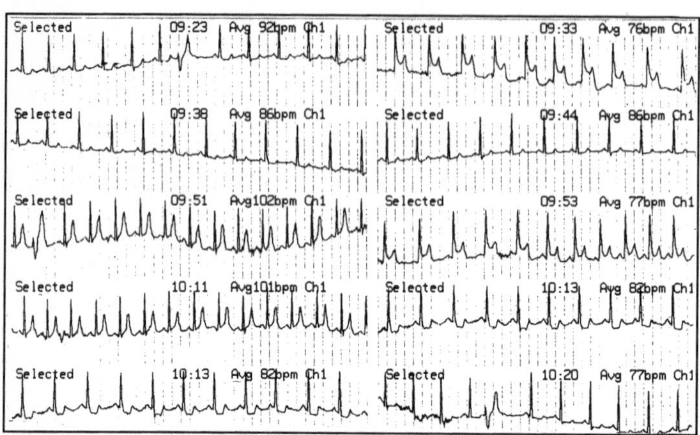

1. What is the diagnosis?

- ❑ A Unstable angina
- ❑ B Crescendo angina
- ❑ C Prinzmetal (variant) angina
- ❑ D Subendocardial infarction
- ❑ E Transmural infarction

Data Interpretation 3 (2 marks)

The following readings are taken from a cardiac catheter of a 14-year-old cyanosed boy:

	Pressure [mmHg]
RA	Mean 6
RV	115/2
PA	22/12
LA	Mean 5
LV	110/0
Aorta	110/60

1. What is the likely diagnosis?

- ❑ A Eisenmenger complex
- ❑ B Pulmonary stenosis
- ❑ C Ebstein's anomaly
- ❑ D Fallot's tetralogy
- ❑ E Ventricular septum defect

Data Interpretation 4 (5 marks)

A 6-year-old girl with short stature is under investigation for hypertension. Auscultation reveals a systolic murmur throughout the precordium with an early systolic click. Cardiac catheterization reveals the following pressures:

	Pressure [mmHg]
RA	Mean 2
RV	25/0
PA	24/8
LA	Mean 5
LV	195/5
Ascending aorta	170/95
Descending aorta	120/60

1. What combination of lesions is present?

❑ A Aortic stenosis and aortic incompetence
❑ B Aortic stenosis and patent ductus arteriosus
❑ C Coarctation and pulmonary incompetence
❑ D Atrial septal defect and aortic stenosis
❑ E Coarctation and bicuspid aortic valve

2. What is your next investigation?

❑ A Growth hormone levels
❑ B Chromosomal analysis
❑ C Hand X-ray
❑ D Urinary 17-ketosteroids
❑ E Combined pituitary function tests

Data Interpretation 5 (4 marks)

A 47-year-old man with familial hypercholesterolaemia is admitted to Coronary Care with 2 mm ST elevation in leads, II, III and aVF. A right-sided cardiac catheter gives the following results:

	Pressure [mmHg]
SVC	Mean 10
RA	Mean 10
RV	19/8
PA	18/5
P. Wedge Pressure	3
Radial artery	95/50

1. What is the likely explanation for these results?

- ❑ A Atrial fibrillation
- ❑ B Complete heart block
- ❑ C Right ventricular infarction
- ❑ D Cardiac tamponade
- ❑ E Septal perforation

Two hours later the patient is found to be in a nodal bradycardia.

2. What does this indicate?

- ❑ A Thrombosis of right coronary artery
- ❑ B Thrombosis of circumflex artery
- ❑ C Re-perfusion injury
- ❑ D Lateral extension of infarct
- ❑ E Apical extension of infarct

Data Interpretation 6 (5 marks)

A 65-year-old pensioner with known ischaemic heart disease is brought to hospital having been found collapsed by the warden. Tablets from his bedside table are presented by the ambulance driver and include aspirin, lisinopril, nitro-glycerine spray, amiloride and phenytoin.

Investigations show:

Na	134 mmol/l
K	5.6 mmol/l
Creatinine	159 μmol/l
Creatinine kinase	8,300 U/l
AST	230 U/l
ALT	56 U/l

ECG: Sinus rhythm 76/min, QRS axis +0°, 2 mm antero-lateral ST depression

1. **What is the likely explanation for these findings?**
2. **What further investigation would you perform?**

Data Interpretation 7 (5 marks)

A 26-year-old woman is admitted to the Coronary Care Unit with suspected endocarditis. The following results are obtained from a right-sided cardiac catheter:

	Pressure [mmHg]	O_2-saturation
RA	Mean 3	71%
RV	28/1	72%
PA	28/15	81%
PCWP	12	-

1. What is the diagnosis?

- ❑ A Atrial septal defect
- ❑ B Ventricular septal defect
- ❑ C Corrected transposition of great arteries
- ❑ D Pulmonary stenosis
- ❑ E Patent ductus arteriosus

2. What definitive therapy would you recommend?

- ❑ A Balloon valvotomy
- ❑ B Surgical correction
- ❑ C Prostaglandin E1
- ❑ D Angiographic embolization
- ❑ E Valve replacement

Data Interpretation 8 (5 marks)

A 56-year-old man is under investigation for increasing shortness of breath on exercise. His chest X-ray shows cardiomegaly and pulmonary congestion. There is no history of chest pain.

The following results are obtained:

Hb	126 g/l
WCC	3.8 x 10^9/l
MCV	101 fl

Echocardiogram:

LV end-systolic volume	150 ml
LV end-diastolic volume	180 ml
Ejection fraction	17%
Moderate mitral regurgitation	

1. What is the likely diagnosis?

- ❑ A Dilating (congestive) cardiomyopathy
- ❑ B Restrictive cardiomyopathy
- ❑ C Hypertrophic cardiomyopathy
- ❑ D Mixed mitral valve disease
- ❑ E Aortic stenosis

2. What is the likely aetiology?

- ❑ A Viral infection
- ❑ B Rheumatic fever
- ❑ C Congenital defect
- ❑ D Endocardial fibrosis
- ❑ E Alcohol abuse

Data Interpretation 9 (4 marks)

The following ECG is recorded during an insurance medical from a 32-year-old builder.

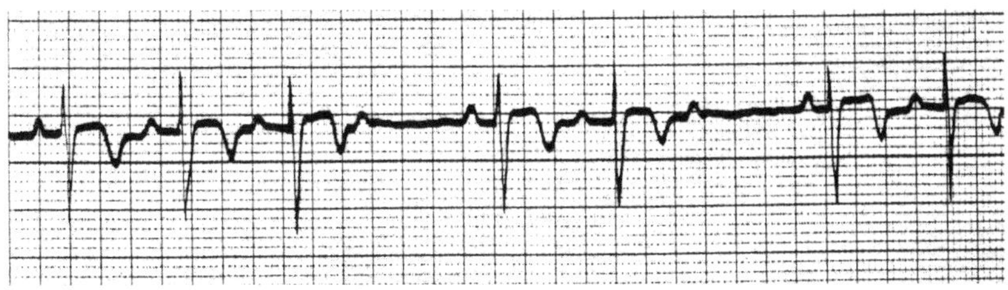

1. What is the diagnosis?

- ❑ A Sick-sinus syndrome
- ❑ B 1° heart block
- ❑ C 2° heart block
- ❑ D 3° heart block
- ❑ E Wandering pacemaker

2. What therapy would you recommend?

- ❑ A Observation only
- ❑ B Atropine
- ❑ C Verapamil
- ❑ D Sotalol
- ❑ E Pacemaker

Data Interpretation 10 (3 marks)

This is the ECG of a 47-year-old man with chest pain.

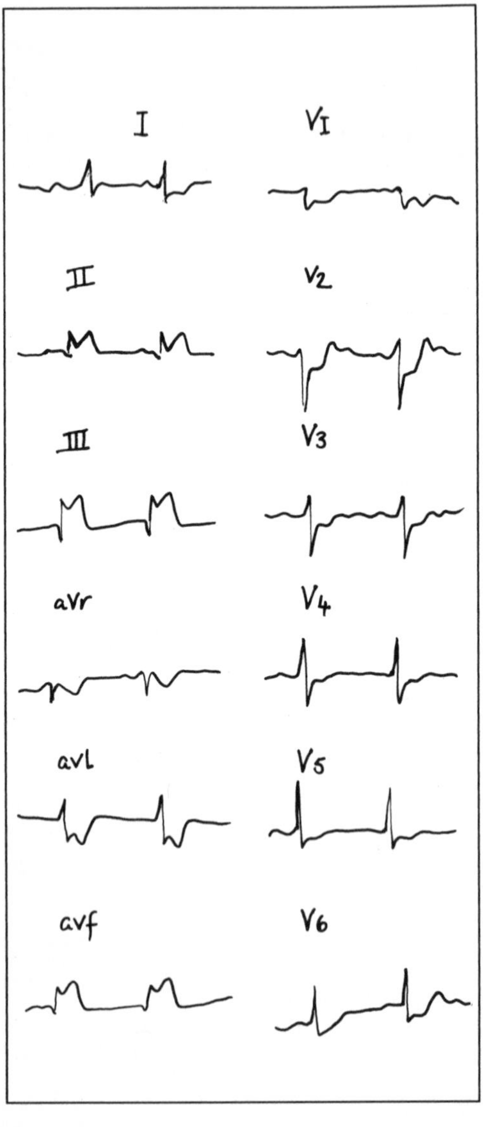

I V1 II V2 III V3 aVr V4 avL V5 avf V6

1. **What does it show?**

Data Interpretation 11 (5 marks)

This is an ECG of a 28-year-old man with intermittent palpitations.

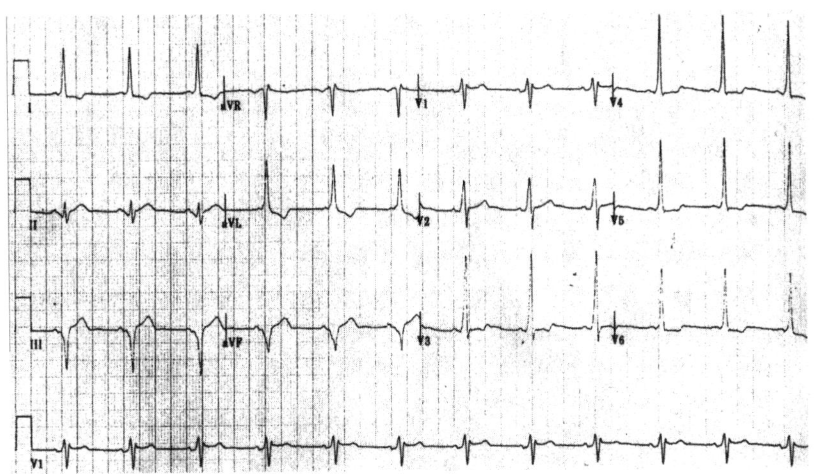

1. What is the diagnosis?

- ❑ A Nodal rhythm
- ❑ B Lone-Ganong-Levine syndrome
- ❑ C Wolff-Parkinson-White Type A
- ❑ D Wolff-Parkinson-White Type B
- ❑ E Bi-fascicular block

2. What is the underlying cause?

- ❑ A Sick-sinus syndrome
- ❑ B Septal ischaemia
- ❑ C Central accessory bundle
- ❑ D Right-sided accessory bundle
- ❑ E Left-sided accessory bundle

Data Interpretation 12 (4 marks)

Following the readings from a cardiac catheter of a 42-year-old woman with worsening dyspnoea.

	Pressure [mmHg]	O_2-saturation
RA	Mean 12	66%
RV	58/10	65%
PA	56/28, Mean 39	64%
LA	Mean 15	95%
LV	120/2	93%
Aorta	120/75	94%

Cardiac output 3.0 l/min.

1. What is the diagnosis?

- ❑ A Hypertrophic obstructive cardiomyopathy
- ❑ B Primary pulmonary hypertension
- ❑ C Mixed aortic valve disease
- ❑ D Mitral stenosis
- ❑ E Ventricular septum defect

2. What complication has arisen?

- ❑ A Shunt reversal
- ❑ B Atrial thrombus
- ❑ C Pulmonary hypertension
- ❑ D Right ventricular dysfunction
- ❑ E Left ventricular infarction

Data Interpretation 13 (6 marks)

A patient is admitted acutely ill, ECG 'A' is recorded on arrival.

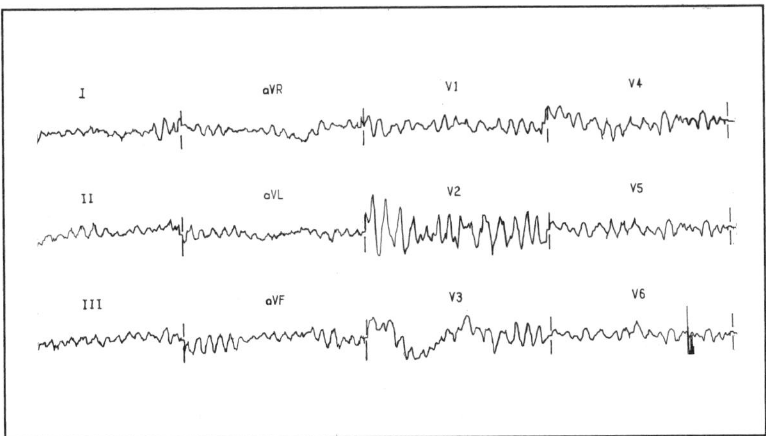

1. **What does it show?**
2. **What is your treatment?**

ECG 'B' is recorded after admission to the Coronary Care Unit.

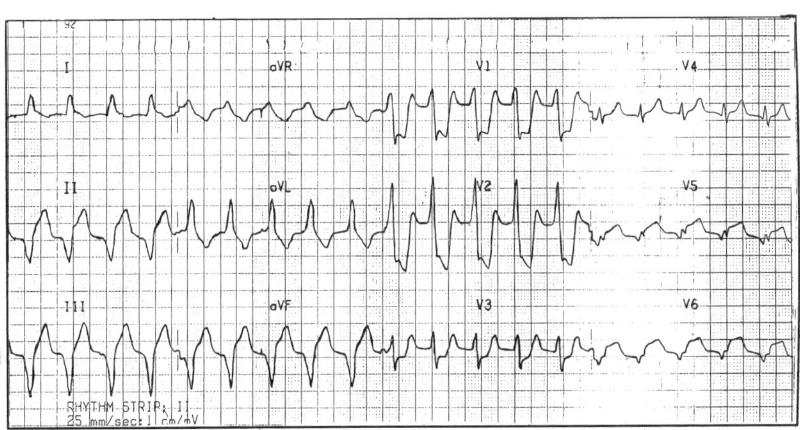

3. **What is the underlying abnormality?**

Data Interpretation 14 (3 marks)

This is the ECG of a 49-year-old woman who has experienced several blackouts over the last 18 months. Pulse 72/min regular, BP 105/85 mmHg in both arms.

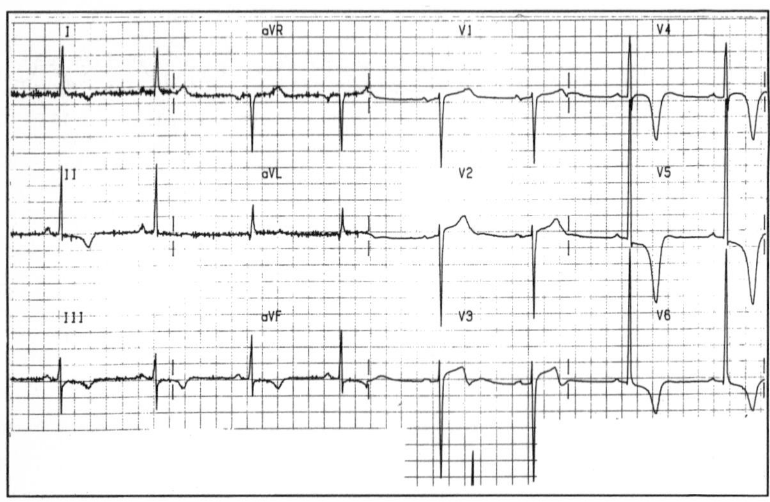

1. What is the most likely diagnosis?

- ☐ A Aortic incompetence
- ☐ B Restrictive cardiomyopathy
- ☐ C Coarctation
- ☐ D Aortic stenosis
- ☐ E Ventricular septum defect

Data Interpretation 15 (2 marks)

A motorcyclist has collided with a bus and is brought into Casualty unconscious. Blood pressure and pulse are unrecordable. The following rhythm strip is obtained:

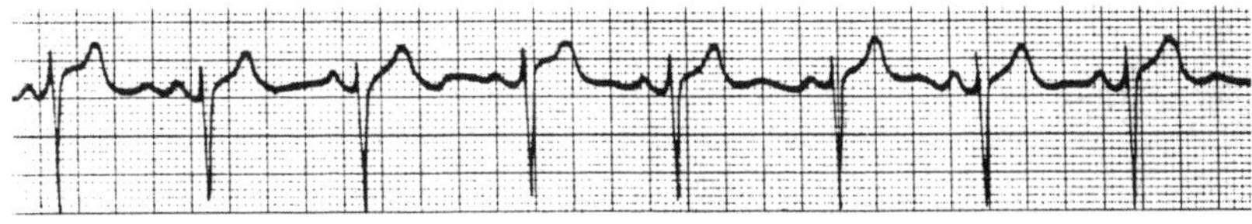

1. **Which of the following injuries is unlikely to account for the findings?**

- ❑ A Serial rib fractures
- ❑ B Aortic rupture
- ❑ C Carotid dissection
- ❑ D Air embolism
- ❑ E Pericardial haemorrhage

Data Interpretation 16 (5 marks)

A 62-year-old smoker is admitted with severe epigastric pain. Pulse 44/min regular, BP 155/65 mmHg.

Creatinine kinase	350 U/l
AST	75 U/l
ESR	28 mm/hr

The following rhythm strip is obtained:

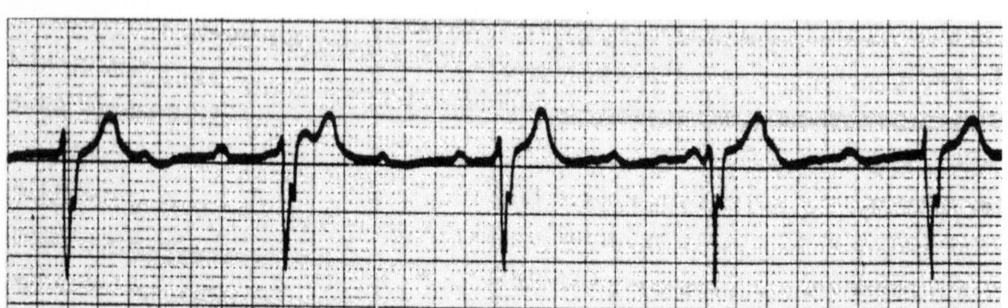

1. **What is the abnormality?**

- ❑ A Left bundle branch block
- ❑ B Sinus bradycardia
- ❑ C Nodal rhythm
- ❑ D 2° atrio-ventricular block
- ❑ E Complete heart block

2. **What is the appropriate management?**

- ❑ A Thrombolysis
- ❑ B Transient pacemaker
- ❑ C External pacemaker
- ❑ D iv atropine
- ❑ E iv heparin

Data Interpretation 17 (5 marks)

A 22-year-old woman presents with amaurosis fugax and a heart murmur. The following are the results of her cardiac catheter study.

	Pressure [mmHg]	O_2 -saturation
SVC	Mean 2	68%
RA	Mean 6	78%
RV	25/2	79%
PA	25/8	80%
LA	Mean 6	97%
LV	110/2	96%
Aorta	110/70	95%

ECG sinus rhythm 64/min, QRS axis +150°, incomplete right bundle branch block.

1. **What is the likely diagnosis?**

- ❑ A Ostium primum atrial septal defect
- ❑ B Patent foramen ovale
- ❑ C Ventricular septum defect
- ❑ D Ostium secundum atrial septal defect
- ❑ E Anomalous pulmonary venous drainage

2. **Which of the following investigations is relatively contra-indicated?**

- ❑ A Ventilation perfusion lung scan
- ❑ B Exercise tolerance test
- ❑ C Coronary angiogram
- ❑ D Cerebral angiogram
- ❑ E Myocardial szintigraphy

Data Interpretation 18 (4 marks)

A 41-year-old man is admitted cold and sweating. The following ECG is taken in the A&E Department.

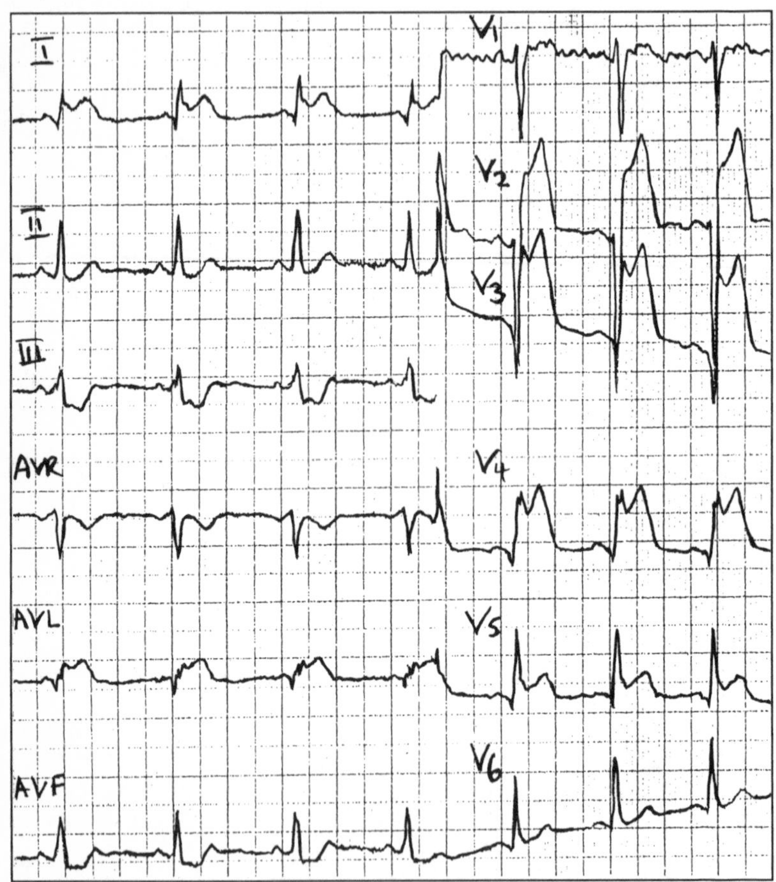

1. Which part of the coronary artery system is affected?

- ❑ A Left anterior descending artery
- ❑ B Left circumflex artery
- ❑ C Posterior descending artery
- ❑ D Left obtuse marginal branch
- ❑ E Left main stem

2. What is the therapy of choice?

- ❑ A Streptokinase and beta-blocker
- ❑ B Urokinase and GTN spray
- ❑ C Aspirin and GTN infusion
- ❑ D Aspirin and r-TPA
- ❑ E iv heparin and GTN spray

Data Interpretation 19 (3 marks)

A 32-year-old woman is investigated for episodes of palpitations and anxiety.

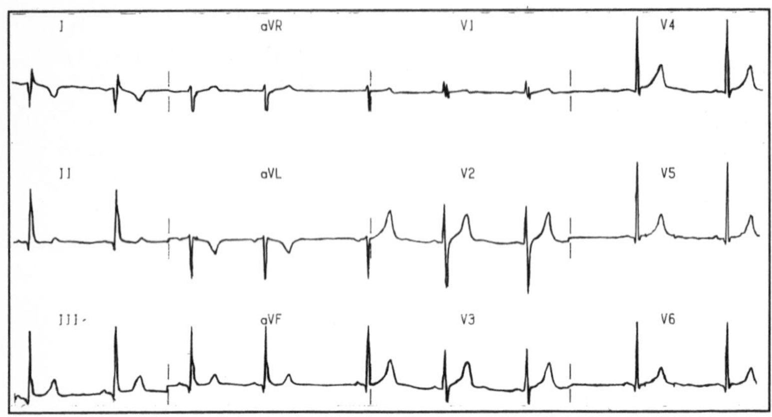

1. **What abnormality does her ECG show?**

Data Interpretation 20 (4 marks)

A 15-year-old thin girl is referred to the Cardiology Department for investigation of palpitations. She also complains of recurrent flank pain.

Arterial blood (on air)	
pH	7.31
O_2	14.0 kPa (105 mmHg)
CO_2	4.0 kPa (30 mmHg)
Bicarbonate	15 mmol/l
Dipstix urine	Blood +, Protein -, Glucose -

ECG: Sinus rhythm 72/min, multi-focal ventricular extrasystoles, QRS axis +75°, descending ST depression in antero-lateral leads, U-waves

1. What is the likely diagnosis?

- ❑ A Chronic liquorice intoxication
- ❑ B Renal tubular acidosis Type I
- ❑ C Fanconi syndrome
- ❑ D Renal tubular acidosis Type II
- ❑ E Anorexia nervosa

2. What is your next investigation?

- ❑ A Abdominal X-ray
- ❑ B 24-hour cardiac monitoring
- ❑ C Intravenous urogram
- ❑ D Echocardiogram
- ❑ E Urine spectroscopy

Data Interpretation 21 (5 marks)

A 43-year-old diabetic is under investigation for deteriorating exercise tolerance. On examination he looks very well, pulse 68/min, regular, BP 160/90 mmHg.

The following results are obtained:

Hb	181 g/l
WCC	5.2 x 10^9/l
Urea & Electrolytes	Normal
Bilirubin	43 mmol/l
AST	412 U/l
ALT	387 U/l

Echocardiogram: Left ventricular dilatation and dyskinesia, ejection fraction 23%

1. What is the cardiac diagnosis?

- ❑ A Ischaemic heart disease
- ❑ B Viral myocarditis
- ❑ C Toxic cardiomyopathy
- ❑ D Amyloidosis
- ❑ E Constrictive pericarditis

2. What therapy would you recommend?

- ❑ A Steroids
- ❑ B Venesection
- ❑ C Cyclophosphamide
- ❑ D α-interferon
- ❑ E Cardiac transplant

Data Interpretation 22 (4 marks)

A 31-year-old Jamaican chef is referred with an 18-month history of shortness of breath. More recently he complained of increased thirst and recurring palpitations. The following rhythm strip is obtained:

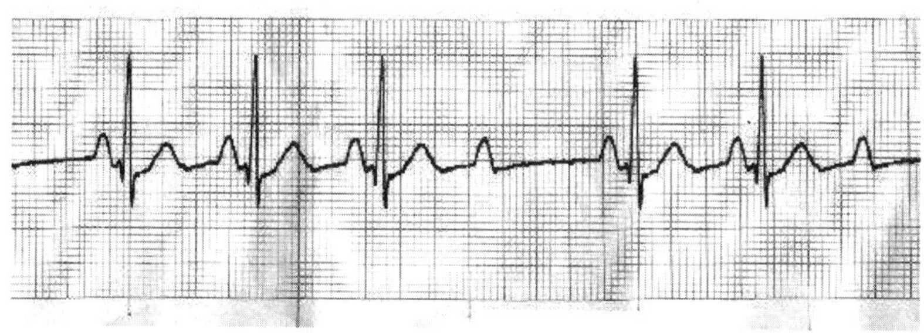

1. What does it show?

- ❑ A Atrial standstill
- ❑ B Sick-sinus syndrome
- ❑ C Mobitz Type 1 heart block
- ❑ D Ectopic atrial pacemaker
- ❑ E Mobitz Type 2 heart block

2. What underlying diagnosis has to be considered?

- ❑ A Kawasaki syndrome
- ❑ B Amyloidosis
- ❑ C Sarcoidosis
- ❑ D Rheumatoid arthritis
- ❑ E Diabetes mellitus

Data Interpretation 23 (5 marks)

An 11-year-old boy is referred for investigation of ataxia and exertional syncope. On examination there is a jerky pulse with an ejection systolic murmur. He also has clawing of the toes and fundoscopy shows temporal pallor of both discs.

Investigations show:

Chest X-ray: Normal
ECG: Left ventricular hypertrophy
Echocardiogram: Septal thickening and mild mitral regurgitation

1. What is the cardiac diagnosis?

- ❑ A Mixed aortic valve disease
- ❑ B Mixed mitral valve disease
- ❑ C Supra-valvar aortic stenosis
- ❑ D Hypertrophic obstructive cardiomyopathy
- ❑ E Cardiac cushion defect

2. What is the underlying condition?

- ❑ A Hereditary sensory motor neuropathy
- ❑ B Friedreich's ataxia
- ❑ C Myotonic dystrophy
- ❑ D Multiple sclerosis
- ❑ E Poliomyelitis

Data Interpretation 24 (3 marks)

The following are the results of a cardiac catheter of a 21-year-old patient with Down's syndrome.

	Pressure [mmHg]	**O_2-saturation**
LA	Mean 8	98%
LV	155/10	90%
Aorta	150/70	91%

1. What is the complete diagnosis?

ENDOCRINOLOGY QUESTIONS: CASE HISTORIES

For 'best-of-five' questions candidates must select one answer only, by putting a cross in the appropriate box.

Case History 1 (9 marks)

A 35-year-old woman presents with a seven-month history of palpitations and intermittent diarrhoea. She describes episodes of 'feeling sweaty and hungry', however has lost 5 kg in weight. She smokes 10 cigarettes a day, drinks approximately 20 units of alcohol per week and her only medication is a low-dose oestrogen contraceptive pill. On examination, she has a pulse rate of 115/min, which is irregular in rate and volume, BP 150/95 mmHg. Examination of the abdomen is normal. Investigations show:

FBC	Normal
U&E's	Normal
Random blood glucose	4.2 mmol/l
Serum albumin	42 g/l
Bilirubin	18 µmol/l
ALT	28 U/l
Total serum thyroxine (tT4)	285 nmol/l (75–150 nmol/l)
3-tri-iodothyronine (fT3)	13.5 pmol/l (3–9 pmol/l)
Serum TSH	9.3 mU/l (0.5–5.5 mU/l)
Serum TRH	Not measurable

Ultrasound of the thyroid shows diffuse enlargement of both lobes and the isthmus without focal abnormality.

1. What is the diagnosis?

❑ A Primary hyperthyroidism
❑ B Secondary hyperthyroidism
❑ C Tertiary hyperthyroidism
❑ D Self-administration of thyroxine
❑ E Subacute thyroiditis

2. Which examination is likely to be the most useful?

- ❑ A TRH test
- ❑ B Ultrasound pelvis
- ❑ C MR scan of pituitary
- ❑ D Thyroid auto-antibodies
- ❑ E Radio-isotope thyroid scan

The patient fails to attend follow-up, but is referred back to the clinic one year later with the following results:

Hb	95 g/l
WCC	1.8 x 10^9/l (89% lymphocytes)
Plt	138 x 10^9/l
Total T4	195 nmol/l (75–150 nmol/l)
Serum TSH	16.2 mU/l (0.5–5.5 mU/l)

3. What therapy has the patient had in the interim?

- ❑ A Radio-iodine therapy
- ❑ B Subtotal thyroidectomy
- ❑ C Partial hypophysectomy
- ❑ D Carbimazole
- ❑ E No treatment

4. What therapy is likely to be most effective?

- ❑ A Carbimazole combined with thyroxine
- ❑ B Total thyroidectomy
- ❑ C Transsphenoidal hypophysectomy
- ❑ D Radiotherapy of pituitary fossa
- ❑ E Propylthiouracil

Case History 2 (10 marks)

A 43-year-old diabetic man is referred for investigation of nocturnal epigastric pain which has been present, on and off, for the last 18 months. He made initial good improvement on ranitidine but has relapsed after seven months. There is a strong family history of diabetes, his father died of carcinoma of the pancreas and his brother has renal stones. The patient is well controlled on intensified insulin therapy and, other than H2-antagonists, he is on no medication. He does not smoke and does not drink alcohol.

A gastroscopy shows a scarred duodenal cap with some active ulceration.

The following blood results are obtained:

Hb	132 g/l
MCV	73 fl
WCC	5.4 x 10^9/l (normal differential)
Plt	231 x 10^9/l
ESR	16 mm/hr
Na	141 mmol/l
K	4.7 mmol/l
Calcium	3.63 mmol/l
Albumin	38 g/l
Liver function tests	Normal
Urinalysis	Normal

An abdominal X-ray shows no evidence of perforation, but bilateral medullary nephrocalcinosis. There are also some erosions in both sacro-iliac joints.

1. What is the likely underlying cause?

- ❑ A Milk-alkali syndrome
- ❑ B Crohn's disease of terminal ileum
- ❑ C Primary hyperparathyroidism
- ❑ D Zollinger-Ellison syndrome
- ❑ E Sarcoidosis

2. What investigation would be the most useful?

- ❑ A Secretin-suppression test
- ❑ B Urease test for Campylobacter
- ❑ C Chest X-ray
- ❑ D Technetium-MIBI-subtraction scan
- ❑ E Small bowel enema

The patient improves initially on proton pump inhibitors, but over the following months develops profuse watery diarrhoea as well as a migrating, scarring rash over the trunk and upper arms. His diabetic control is worsening, he is also complaining of headaches and, on examination, a bi-temporal hemianopia is found.

3. Suggest two further tests

- ❑ A MR pituitary and CT pancreas
- ❑ B CT brain and small bowel enema
- ❑ C Combined pituitary function tests and radio-labelled white cell scan
- ❑ D Stool cultures and lumbar puncture
- ❑ E Small bowel biopsy and visual evoked potentials

4. What is the unifying diagnosis?

- ❑ A Gardner's syndrome
- ❑ B Peutz-Jegher's syndrome
- ❑ C Wermer syndrome (multiple endocrine neoplasia Type I)
- ❑ D Verner-Morrison syndrome (pancreatic vipoma)
- ❑ E Sipple syndrome (multiple endocrine neoplasia Type IIa)

5. What is the association with the skin rash?

- ❑ A Pancreatic vipoma
- ❑ B Small bowel adenocarcinoma
- ❑ C Phaeochromocytoma
- ❑ D Glucagonoma
- ❑ E Parathyroid adenoma

Case History 3 (9 marks)

A 56-year-old butcher presents with an eight month history of malaise, headaches, depression and backache. He has also found it difficult climbing the stairs at home and getting out of his car. He was previously healthy, smokes 25 cigarettes a day but does not drink alcohol. His only medication is diclofenac for back pain. On examination, he has a plethoric face, and multiple ecchymoses are present within the skin of arms and abdomen. There is truncal obesity and striae are present over the abdomen.

There is some proximal muscle wasting, but no fasciculation and the reflexes are present.

Blood pressure is 190/105 mmHg and he has Grade II hypertensive retinopathy. Investigations show:

Hb	159 g/l
WCC	7.8 x 10^9/l
Plt	238 x 10^9/l
Na	146 mmol/l
K	3.1 mmol/l
Creatinine	92 μmol/l

Oral glucose tolerance test					
Time [minutes]	**0**	**30**	**60**	**90**	**120**
Glucose [mmol/l]	6.9	8.5	11.2	9.8	8.9
Growth hormone [mU/l]	6.2 (2–8 mU/l)	4.8	4.5	3.9	2.8

1. What do these results imply?

- ❑ A Impaired glucose tolerance
- ❑ B Acromegaly
- ❑ C Manifest diabetes mellitus
- ❑ D Chronic liver disease
- ❑ E Pituitary dysfunction

A morning blood sample shows the following result:
09.00 a.m. Cortisol 899 nmol/l (200–700 nmol/l)

After two days of 2 mg/day dexamethasone, the following result is obtained:

09.00 a.m.	Cortisol	801 nmol/l

Then after a further two days of 8 mg/day dexamethasone:

09.00 a.m.	Cortisol	769 nmol/l

2. Which of the following two differential diagnoses are consistent with these results?

- ❑ A Pituitary adenoma and adrenal carcinoma
- ❑ B Hyperthalamic dysfunction and pituitary adenoma
- ❑ C Adrenal adenoma and ectopic ACTH secretion
- ❑ D Factitious administration of cortisol and pituitary adenoma
- ❑ E Bronchial carcinoma and Cushing's disease

3. Which of the following tests is most likely to differentiate between the two?

- ❑ A Insulin stress test
- ❑ B Renal ultrasound scan
- ❑ C CRH test
- ❑ D MR scan of the pituitary
- ❑ E Serum ACTH levels

Following surgical treatment, the patient becomes hypotensive and oliguric. Examination of the abdomen reveals peritonism with absent bowel sounds. The following results are obtained:

Na	131 mmol/l
K	5.8 mmol/l
Urea	18.6 mmol/l
Creatinine	256 µmol/l

4. What complication has developed?

- ❑ A Acute pituitary failure
- ❑ B Acute tubular necrosis
- ❑ C Acute adrenal failure
- ❑ D Acute hydrocephalus
- ❑ E Waterhouse-Friderichsen syndrome

Case History 4 (8 marks)

A 69-year-old woman presents with weight loss, polyuria and polydipsia. She complains of upper abdominal and back pain and has lost 3 kg in weight. She is a lifelong non-smoker, drinks one glass of sherry a night and her only medication is bendrofluazide 2.5 mg for hypertension. On examination, she is pale, pulse 72/min regular, BP 155/90 mmHg. Her apex beat is displaced into the anterior axillary line and there are fine crackles at both lung bases. She is tender in the epigastrium, but there is no palpable enlargement of liver or spleen and no lymph nodes can be felt.

Blood results:

Hb	121 g/l
WCC	3.2 x 10^9/l
Plt	105 x 10^9/l
ESR	28 mm/hr

The blood film shows a small number of nucleated red cells and myeloblasts.

Na	138 mmol/l
K	3.3 mmol/l
Urea	9.8 mmol/l
Calcium	3.7 mmol/l
Phosphate	1.4 mmol/l (0.75–1.5 mmol/l)
Bilirubin	18 µmol/l
Alk. phosphatase	180 U/l (20–120 U/l)
Albumin	38 g/l
Total protein	62 g/l

The patient is given 40 mg hydrocortisone x 3/day for 10 days.

Calcium	3.1 mmol/l

1. What further investigation would you recommend?

- ❑ A Abdominal X-ray
- ❑ B Parathormone levels
- ❑ C Radio-isotope bone scan
- ❑ D Ultrasound scan of the neck
- ❑ E Immune electrophoresis

2. What is the likely diagnosis?

- ❑ A Primary hyperparathyroidism
- ❑ B Sarcoidosis
- ❑ C Ectopic PTH secretion
- ❑ D Metastatic carcinoma
- ❑ E Myeloma

3. How do you interpret the blood film?

- ❑ A Leukoerythroblastic film due to marrow invasion
- ❑ B Myelofibrosis
- ❑ C Myelodysplasia
- ❑ D Aplastic anaemia
- ❑ E Rebound phenomenon

4. What initial management do you suggest?

- ❑ A iv saline
- ❑ B High-dose systemic steroids
- ❑ C Chlorambucil
- ❑ D Parathyroid injection with alcohol
- ❑ E Radiotherapy of primary tumour

Case History 5 (10 marks)

A 71-year-old retired carpenter is admitted to the Casualty Department following a grand mal fit. In the resuscitation room the patient has two further generalised seizures without regaining consciousness between them. His past medical history includes hypertension, which has been well controlled over the last 15 years on Moduretic® (amiloride and hydrochlorothiazide). A year previously his diet-controlled diabetes worsened and he was started on chlorpropamide by his GP.

On examination, the patient has a Glasgow Coma Scale of 7/15, only localising to pain. There is mild meningism but no focal neurology. Fundoscopy only shows some silver wiring and AV-nipping. The chest is clear and examination of heart and abdomen are normal. The following results are obtained:

Hb	146 g/l
WCC	10.6 x 10^9/l
Plt	285 x 10^9/l
Na	110 mmol/l
K	3.5 mmol/l
Urea	4.0 mmol/l
Creatinine	168 μmol/l
Glucose	9 mmol/l
Urine osmolality	589 mosm/kg
Chest X-ray	normal
CT brain	normal

1. What is the serum osmolality?

- ❑ A 230
- ❑ B 240
- ❑ C 253.5
- ❑ D 267
- ❑ E 270.5

2. What is the likely diagnosis?

- ❑ A Water intoxication
- ❑ B Peripheral diabetes insipidus
- ❑ C Central diabetes insipidus
- ❑ D Addisonian crisis
- ❑ E Inappropriate ADH secretion

3. What two treatments would you instigate?

- ❑ A iv saline and phenobarbitone
- ❑ B iv hydrocortisone and diazepam
- ❑ C im hydrocortisone and iv frusemide
- ❑ D Fluid restriction and iv diazepam
- ❑ E iv phenytoin and saline

No medical bed is available and the patient is treated by the A&E staff. The following morning the patient is transferred under your care. He has made an initial recovery, his Glasgow Coma Scale returning to 14, with some remaining disorientation. However, over the following hours the patient deteriorates rapidly again and becomes hypotensive and unresponsive. There is generalised reduction in tone but both plantars are up-going.

Biochemical profile now reveals:

Na	129 mmol/l
K	2.8 mmol/l
Urea	2.2 mmol/l
Creatinine	151 µmol/l
Glucose	8 mmol/l

4. What is the likely cause?

- ❑ A Diazepam overdose
- ❑ B Central pontine myelinolysis
- ❑ C Cerebral oedema
- ❑ D Cerebral infarction
- ❑ E Brain stem haemorrhage

5. What examination is most likely to be diagnostic?

- ❑ A CT brain
- ❑ B MR brain
- ❑ C EEG
- ❑ D ADH levels
- ❑ E Urinary electrolytes

Case History 6 (8 marks)

A 35-year-old woman presents with malaise and increasing shortness of breath. Since the birth of her second child three years ago her periods have been irregular with intermittent menorrhagia and she has gained five kilos in weight. She has been diagnosed as having post-natal depression and she has lost her job as a secretary. On examination, she is pale and mildly tachypnoeic. Her heart sounds are quiet without any murmurs, her chest is clear. Pulse 56/min, BP 115/60 mmHg.

Examination of the CNS reveals a mild reduction in the lateral visual field of the right eye. Both ankle jerks are sluggish.

Investigations:

Hb	103 g/l
MCV	100 fl
WCC	4.1 x 10^9/l (normal differential)
Plt	273 x 10^9/l
Na	141 mmol/l
K	4.2 mmol/l
Creatinine	88 µmol/l
Total T4	34 nmol/l (75–150 nmol/l)
Free T3	1.5 pmol/l (3–9 pmol/l)
Serum TSH	58 mu/l (0.5–5.5 mu/l)
9am plasma cortisol	280 nmol/l (200–700 nmol/l)
Prolactin	3,750 U/l (< 700 units/l)
Gonadotrophins	Normal

Thyroid, microsomal and thyroglobulin autoantibodies positive

ECG: sinus bradycardia with low voltage complexes.

1. **What is the diagnosis?**

- ❑ A Sheehan syndrome (pituitary infarction)
- ❑ B Primary hypothyroidism
- ❑ C Prolactinoma
- ❑ D Non-functioning pituitary adenoma
- ❑ E Subacute thyroiditis

2. What investigation would you perform next?

- ❑ A Combined pituitary function tests
- ❑ B Lateral skull X-ray
- ❑ C Viral serology
- ❑ D Ultrasound of thyroid
- ❑ E MR scan of pituitary

3. What is the cause of the raised prolactin levels?

- ❑ A Increased TRH production
- ❑ B Pituitary tumour
- ❑ C Pituitary failure
- ❑ D Hypothalamic failure
- ❑ E Pregnancy

4. What is the treatment?

- ❑ A Oral steroids
- ❑ B Radio-iodine therapy
- ❑ C Oral thyroxine
- ❑ D Transsphenoidal hypophysectomy
- ❑ E Oral bromocriptine

Case History 7 (13 marks)

A 13-year-old girl is under investigation for tall stature, absent development of breasts and male distribution of pubic and body hair. She has never had a period and has recently developed hypertension. On examination, she is found to be on the 95th percentile for height and the 50th percentile for weight. No significant breast development is present, but there is hypertrophy of the clitoris and the labia majora. Her BP is 175/95 mmHg, pulse 88/min, regular, and examination of chest and cardiovascular system is otherwise unremarkable. No focal neurology.

The following results are obtained:

FBC	Normal
Na	149 mmol/l
K	3.4 mmol/l
Urea	7.2 mmol/l
Creatinine	129 μmol/l
Albumin	42 g/l
Luteinizing hormone	< 0.1 U/l (2.5–15 U/l)
FSH	< 0.1 U/l (0.3–3.0 U/l)
Testosterone	10.7 nmol/l (< 2.0 nmol/l)
9am cortisol	23 nmol/l (100–700 nmol/l)
Urinary 11-deoxycorticosterone	4.3 μg/24hrs (0.1–0.4 μg/24hrs)
Plasma renin	16 pmol/l (85–410 pmol/l)

1. **What is the diagnosis?**
2. **Why is the patient hypertensive?**
3. **What is the likelihood of this patient being diabetic?**
4. **What is the treatment?**

Case History 8 (7 marks)

A 6-year-old boy presents with a generalised seizure to his GP and is referred to the endocrine clinic for investigation of hypocalcaemia. There is a weak family history of 'bone problems' of which his paternal grandfather was diagnosed at the age of 12.

On examination, the patient is on the 25th percentile for height and shows swelling of most large joints and the costo-sternal junction. Trousseau and Chvosteck's signs are positive. Mental development is normal for age. No soft tissue calcifications are seen. He has always been on an healthy diet, has no prolonged episodes of diarrhoea and took no regular medication.

Blood results show:

Hb	146 g/l
WCC	4.2 x 10^9/l
Plt	173 x 10^9/l
ESR	6 mm/h
Na	139 mmol/l
K	4.1 mmol/l
Calcium	1.8 mmol/l
Phosphate	0.45 mmol/l
Creatinine	55 µmol/l
Bilirubin	12 µmol/l
Alkaline phosphatase	761 U/l
Parathormone	273 pmol/l (10–90 pmol/l)

X-ray of his hands show widened growth plates with cupped and frayed metaphyses.

1. **What is the most likely diagnosis?**
2. **How would you confirm it?**
3. **What is the likely inheritance based on the information given?**

ENDOCRINOLOGY QUESTIONS: DATA INTERPRETATIONS

For 'best-of-five' questions candidates must select one answer only, by putting a cross in the appropriate box.

Data Interpretation 1 (2 marks)

A 14-year-old girl with short stature is under investigation for delayed skeletal maturation. The following results were obtained during an Ellsworth-Howard test.

	Baseline	**After infusion of parathormone**
Urinary phosphate [nmol/d]	4.8	5.0
Urinary cyclic-AMP [nmol/mmol creatinine]	0.31	0.29
Parathyroid hormone [pmol/l]	261 (10–90)	
9am growth hormone [mU/l]	7 (4–8)	

1. **What is the likely diagnosis?**

- ❑ A Hypoparathyroidism
- ❑ B Hyperparathyroidism
- ❑ C Pseudohypoparathyroidism Type I
- ❑ D Pseudohypoparathyroidism Type II
- ❑ E Pseudo-pseudohypoparathyroidism

Data Interpretation 2 (2 marks)

A 34-year-old nurse is under investigation for weight loss, episodes of early morning dizziness and faints. The following results were obtained after an overnight fast:

Plasma glucose	2.3 mmol/l
Plasma insulin	460 pmol/l (35–150 pmol/l)
C-peptide	0.15 nmol/l (0.2–0.6 nmol/l)

1. What is the likely diagnosis?

- ❑ A Insulinoma
- ❑ B Glucagonoma
- ❑ C Self-administration of insulin
- ❑ D Self-administration of sulphonylureas
- ❑ E Acromegaly

Data Interpretation 3 (5 marks)

A 56-year-old man presents with headaches and hypertension. The following results were obtained during an oral glucose tolerance test (75 gms of oral glucose equivalent):

Time [minutes]	Plasma glucose [mmol/l]	Growth hormone [mU/l]
0	8.9	12
30	12.8	18
60	14.4	28
90	13.8	34
120	12.2	23

Prolactin 1,680 mU/l (75-350 mU/l)

1. What is the underlying diagnosis?

- ❑ A Diabetes mellitus
- ❑ B Prolactinoma
- ❑ C Multiple endocrine neoplasia Type I
- ❑ D Multiple endocrine neoplasia Type II
- ❑ E Acromegaly

2. What complication has developed?

- ❑ A Impaired glucose tolerance
- ❑ B Malignant glucagonoma
- ❑ C Pituitary failure
- ❑ D Compression of pituitary stalk
- ❑ E Hyperthalamic failure

Data Interpretation 4 (4 marks)

A 23-year-old man is under investigation for significantly taller stature than his parents. He is 1.93 m tall with an arm span of 1.97 m. Pubis to heel distance 99 cm, pubis to vertex 95 cm. The metacarpal index estimated on a hand X-ray indicates arachnodactyly.

Blood results show:

Testosterone	4.6 nmol/l (10–30 nmol/l)
Luteinizing hormone	28 U/l (< 6 U/l)
Follicle stimulating hormone	43 U/l (< 6 U/l)

Buccal Smear: Barr bodies present

1. What is the diagnosis?

- ❑ A Turner's syndrome
- ❑ B Klinefelter's syndrome
- ❑ C Noonan's syndrome
- ❑ D Marfan's syndrome
- ❑ E Testicular feminization

2. What management is appropriate?

- ❑ A Family screening
- ❑ B Testicular biopsy
- ❑ C MR scan of pituitary
- ❑ D Combined pituitary function test
- ❑ E Testosterone replacement

Data Interpretation 5 (4 marks)

A 25-year-old women presents with atrial fibrillation. The only medication she is taking is the oral contraceptive pill.

Investigations show:

Total T4	164 nmol/l (70–150 nmol/l)
Free T4	14.2 pmol/l (10–25 pmol/l)

A TRH test is performed
TSH levels after 20 μg TRH iv:

0 minutes	< 0.1 U/l
30 minutes	< 0.1 U/l

1. **What is the diagnosis?**
2. **How do you interpret the total T4 level?**

Data Interpretation 6 (4 marks)

A 38-year-old in-patient on a psychiatric unit is investigated for polydipsia and polyuria. A water deprivation test is performed.

Time [hours]	0	2	5	8
Plasma osmolality [mosm/kg]	289	302	307	309
Urine osmolality [mosm/kg]	121	134	159	188

1. What is the likely underlying diagnosis?

- ❑ A Psychogenic polydipsia
- ❑ B Central diabetes insipidus
- ❑ C Psychogenic water deprivation
- ❑ D Peripheral diabetes insipidus
- ❑ E Renal tubular acidosis Type II

2. What would you expect after the im injection of DDAVP (Vasopressin)?

- ❑ A No change
- ❑ B Increase in urine osmolality > 15%
- ❑ C Drop in plasma osmolality > 10 mosmol/kg
- ❑ D Increase in plasma osmolality > 10%
- ❑ E Rise in urine osmolality > 500 mosmol/kg

Data Interpretation 7 (3 marks)

The following results were obtained during an insurance medical examination of a 48-year-old manager:

Na	138 mmol/l
K	4.1 mmol/l
Creatinine	92 µmol/l
Calcium	2.86 mmol/l
Phosphate	0.85 mmol/l
Alkaline phosphatase	99 U/l
Magnesium	1.3 mmol/l (0.7–1.0 mmol/l)
Parathormone	0.3 pmol/l (1.5–6.5 pmol/l)
Urinary calcium	0.9 mmol/24h (2.5–6 mmol/24h)

1. What is the diagnosis?

- ❑ A Milk-alkali syndrome
- ❑ B Sarcoidosis
- ❑ C Renal tubular acidosis Type I
- ❑ D Familial hypocalciuric hypercalcaemia
- ❑ E Paget's disease

Data Interpretation 8 (5 marks)

A 49-year-old man is under investigation for hypertension, he has a two month history of malaise and weight loss, and has recently developed dysphagia. The following blood results are obtained:

Na	144 mmol/l
K	4.2 mmol/l
Urea	11.8 mmol/l
Calcium	2.9 mmol/l
Phosphate	0.4 mmol/l

A radio-isotope bone scan shows no evidence of metastases. 24-hour blood pressure monitoring shows sustained hypertension between 170/95 to 195/105 mmHg.

1. **Suggest two further investigations.**
2. **What is the likely diagnosis?**

Data Interpretation 9 (6 marks)

A 42-year-old woman presents with a tender neck swelling. The following results are obtained:

Hb	144 g/l
WCC	5.2 x 10^9/l
ESR	99 mm/h
Total T4	192 pmol/l (75–150 pmol/l)
TSH	<0.1 mU/l (0.5–5.5 mU/l)

^{99m}Technetium thyroid scan shows diffuse reduction in uptake, no hot spots.

1. What is the most likely diagnosis?

- ❑ A Subacute thyroiditis
- ❑ B Acute bacterial thyroiditis
- ❑ C Auto-immune thyroiditis
- ❑ D Iodine deficiency
- ❑ E Toxic multi-nodular goitre

2. What management is most appropriate?

- ❑ A Ultrasound scan and antibiotics
- ❑ B Thyroid antibodies and oral thyroxine
- ❑ C Fine needle aspirate and systemic steroids
- ❑ D Estimation of free T3 and T4 and carbimazole
- ❑ E Radio-iodine therapy and oral thyroxine

3. What is the most likely complication without treatment?

- ❑ A Abscess formation
- ❑ B Established thyrotoxicosis
- ❑ C Malignant change
- ❑ D Hypothyroidism
- ❑ E Solid fibrosis of the thyroid

Data Interpretation 10 (5 marks)

A 42-year-old woman presents with secondary amenorrhoea, malaise and anaemia. The following are the results after the combined administration of 0.15 μ/kg of insulin, 200 μg TRH and 100 μg GN-releasing hormone.

Time [min]	0	30	60	120
Glucose [mmol/l]	4.4	1.9	2.1	6.8
GH [mU/l]	2.5 (< 10)	4.8	9.2 (>20)	7.9
TSH [mU/l]	4.2 (5-20)	5.7	4.1	
Prolactin [mU/l]	5,320 (100-55)	5,820	5,950	
LH [mU/l]	1.5 (2-4)	13.8 (15-30)	3.2	

1. **What two diagnoses can be made from these results?**
2. **What is your next investigation?**

Data Interpretation 11 (5 marks)

A 50-year-old male presents with malaise and dizzy spells. These are his results after 250 μg tetracosactrin.

Cortisol at 0 minutes	128 nmol/l
Cortisol at 30 minutes	261 nmol/l
Cortisol at 60 minutes	301 nmol/l

1. What diagnosis is excluded by these results?

❑ A Addison's disease
❑ B Long-term steroid therapy
❑ C Pituitary failure
❑ D Cushing's syndrome
❑ E Hypothalamic failure

Following the short synacthen® test, the patient is given 1 mg of depot tetracosactrin im
Cortisol after 24 hours 612 nmol/l

2. What diagnosis is consistent with these results?

❑ A Addison's disease
❑ B Adrenal carcinoma
❑ C Cushing's syndrome
❑ D Nelson's syndrome
❑ E Long-term steroid therapy

Data Interpretation 12 (5 marks)

A 15-year-old boy is under investigation for the following blood results:

Na	136 mmol/l
K	3.2 mmol/l
Urea	6.1 mmol/l
Creatinine	62 μmol/l
Bicarbonate	21 mmol/l
Calcium	2.1 mmol/l
Albumin	41 g/l
Urine pH	6.9

After oral administration of 100 mg/kg ammonium chloride, the following results are obtained:

Time [min]	**0**	**120**
Serum bicarbonate [mmol/l]	23	15
Urine pH	6.1	5.8

1. What is the most likely diagnosis?

- ❑ A Lactic acidosis
- ❑ B Renal tubular acidosis Type I
- ❑ C Renal tubular acidosis Type II
- ❑ D Cystinuria
- ❑ E Alport's syndrome

2. What investigation would be the most useful?

- ❑ A Plain abdominal radiograph
- ❑ B Urinary calcium excretion
- ❑ C Urinary protein electrophoresis
- ❑ D Renal biopsy
- ❑ E Renal ultrasound scan

Data Interpretation 13 (5 marks)

A 61-year-old woman is under investigation for a six-month history of tiredness and weight loss. These are her blood results:

Na	132 mmol/l
K	5.8 mmol/l
Urea	5.7 mmol/l
Creatinine	138 µmol/l
Hb	107 g/l
MCV	105 fl
WCC	3.8 x 10^9/l
Plt	158 x 10^9/l
TSH	9.8 mU/l (0.5–5.5 mU/l)
9am cortisol	66 nmol/l
9am growth hormone	6 mU/l (4–10 mU/l)

1. What is the diagnosis?

- ❑ A Sheehan's syndrome
- ❑ B Addison's disease
- ❑ C Polyglandular failure (Schmidt's syndrome)
- ❑ D Hashimoto's thyroiditis
- ❑ E Acromegaly

2. Which of the following investigations would be the most useful?

- ❑ A Auto-antibody screen
- ❑ B MR scan of pituitary
- ❑ C Short synacthen test
- ❑ D TRH test
- ❑ E Ultrasound scan thyroid

Data Interpretation 14 (6 marks)

A 54-year-old publican presents with a hoarse voice and an increasing inability to climb stairs and get out of his chair. The weakness worsens throughout the day. Investigations show:

Na	144 mmol/l
K	2.9 mmol/l
Urea	3.7 mmol/l
Glucose	13.2 mmol/l
Bicarbonate	34 mmol/l
Random cortisol	985 nmol/l

1. **Suggest two further investigations.**
2. **Give two possible reasons for the myopathy.**

Data Interpretation 15 (5 marks)

A 26-year-old woman is under investigation for oligomenorrhoea and primary infertility. Blood results are as follows:

Na	134 mmol/l
K	4.1 mmol/l
Creatinine	94 µmol/l
Testosterone	2.7 nmol/l (0.8–1.6 nmol/l)
Follicle stimulating hormone	6 U/l (< 8 U/l in follicular phase)
Luteinizing hormone	23 U/l (< 6 U/l in follicular phase)
7-hydroxyprogesterone	2.8 nmol/l (< 15 nmol/l)

1. What diagnosis is the most likely?

- ❑ A Testicular feminization
- ❑ B Cushing's syndrome
- ❑ C Congenital adrenal hyperplasia
- ❑ D Polycystic ovary syndrome
- ❑ E Primary ovarian failure

2. What investigation would be the most helpful?

- ❑ A Urinary free cortisol
- ❑ B Urinary 17-corticosteroids
- ❑ C Ultrasound scan pelvis
- ❑ D Chromosomal analysis
- ❑ E Gonadotrophin-releasing hormone (GN-RH) test

Data Interpretation 16 (5 marks)

A 15-year-old boy is sent to the endocrine clinic for investigation of short stature and obesity. He has underdeveloped genitals, but normal intellectual development. The following blood results are obtained:

Na	140 mmol/l
K	5.0 mmol/l
Urea	8.5 mmol/l
Creatinine	112 µmol/l
Glucose	6.5 mmol/l
Testosterone	2.5 nmol/l (pre-puberty 1–4 nmol/l, post-puberty 12–30 nmol/l)
Urine osmolality	242 mosmol/kg

After administration of 100 µg gonadotrophin-releasing hormone (GN-RH), the following results are obtained:

Time [mins]	0	30	60	120
LH [U/l]	1.5 (1-10)	1.8	3.2 (10-50)	17.3
FSH [U/l]	0.3 (1-5)	0.8	1.2 (1-7)	7.4

1. What does the GN-RH test indicate?

- ❑ A Hypogonadotrophic hypogonadism
- ❑ B Hypergonadotrophic hypogonadism
- ❑ C Pituitary failure
- ❑ D Testicular failure
- ❑ E Androgen resistance

2. What is the likely underlying diagnosis?

- ❑ A Noonan's syndrome
- ❑ B Kallmann's syndrome
- ❑ C Craniopharyngioma
- ❑ D Klinefelter's syndrome
- ❑ E Constitutional delay

GASTROENTEROLOGY QUESTIONS: CASE HISTORIES

For 'best-of-five' questions candidates must select one answer only, by putting a cross in the appropriate box.

Case History 1 (8 marks)

A 23-year-old male travel agent presents to his GP with a short history of increasing heartburn and dysphagia. He was treated with moderate success with anti-reflux medication, but over the following months developed recurring episodes of spasmodic abdominal pain associated with watery diarrhoea. He has lost 2 kg in weight, there is cervical lymphadenopathy, abdominal examination is unremarkable. Two dark nodules are present on his arm. The following results are obtained:

Hb	122 g/l
MCV	98/fl
WBC	3.8 x 10^9/l
Plt	156 x 10^9/l
ESR	18 mm/hr
Electrolytes	Normal
LFTs	Normal
Albumin	28 g/l
Faecal occult blood x 3 -ve	

A Dicopac® test shows the following results:

Urinary excretion of B_{12}	15%
Urinary excretion of combined intrinsic factor and B_{12}	19%

1. What do these results suggest?

- ❑ A Normal B_{12} metabolism
- ❑ B Pernicious anaemia
- ❑ C Terminal ileal disease
- ❑ D Atrophic gastritis
- ❑ E Bacterial overgrowth

The patient is admitted for investigations. A barium swallow shows fine confluent ulceration of the oesophagus. Colonoscopy shows small patches of inflammation in the large bowel. The ileo-caecal junction shows nodular thickening of the bowel wall, the mucosa is intact except for a few small areas of aphthous ulceration.

2. What is the likely cause for the patient's dysphagia?

- ❑ A Barrett's oesophagus
- ❑ B Candida
- ❑ C Cytomegaly virus
- ❑ D Plummer-Vinson syndrome
- ❑ E Gastro-oesophageal reflux

3. What is the likely underlying cause?

- ❑ A Ulcerative colitis
- ❑ B Crohn's disease
- ❑ C HIV infection
- ❑ D Campylobacter infection
- ❑ E Small bowel carcinoma

An ultrasound of the abdomen shows several hypoechoic foci in the liver and mild splenomegaly. An indolent mass is seen in the right iliac fossa.

4. What complication has occurred?

- ❑ A Haematogenic liver abscesses
- ❑ B Adenocarcinoma with liver metastases
- ❑ C Focal fatty change due to malabsorption
- ❑ D Hepatoma
- ❑ E Secondary lymphoma

Case History 2 (6 marks)

A 38-year-old man living in shared accommodation is brought to the A&E Department pyrexial and obtunded. Over the last ten days he has complained of malaise, headaches and 'pains all over'. He has become confused and has been incontinent with several episodes of diarrhoea. He is a smoker of 30 per day, drinks 40–50 units of alcohol per week and works part-time for the local water company.

On examination the patient is jaundiced, with a temperature of 39.2°C. He has a regular tachycardia of 116/min, Blood pressure 105/65 mmHg, normal heart sounds. There is two finger tender hepatomegaly, the tip of the spleen can just be palpated under the left costal margin. The patient shows mild photophobia and neck stiffness, but Kernig's sign is negative and there is no focal neurology. Fundoscopy is normal. Some petechial haemorrhages are present over the trunk and the thighs.

The following results are obtained:

Hb	119 g/l
MCV	96 fl
WBC	19 x 10^9/l (95% neutrophils)
Plt	98 x 10^8/l
Prothrombin time	19 s (control 13 s)
APTT	46 s (control < 34 s)
Na	133 mmol/l
K	5.1 mmol/l
Urea	19.5 mmol/l
Creatinine	205 µmol/l
Bilirubin	92 µmol/l
Albumin	32 g/l
Dipstix urine	Blood +++, Bilirubin +++, Protein ++

1. What two investigations would be most useful

❑ A ECG and Chest X-ray
❑ B Ultrasound abdomen and liver biopsy
❑ C Blood cultures and urine serology
❑ D Enhanced CT brain and lumbar puncture
❑ E CT abdomen and renal biopsy

2. What is the likely diagnosis?

❑ A Leptospirosis
❑ B Bacterial meningitis
❑ C Herpes simplex encephalitis
❑ D Brucellosis
❑ E Shigellosis

Case History 3 (8 marks)

A 36-year-old marathon runner presents to his GP with an itchy rash over both elbows. He has also noticed a slight decrease in his exercise tolerance, but otherwise feels well. On examination he is 180 cm tall, weighing 61 kg. Over the last few months he has noticed recurrent painful lesions in his mouth. The patient is taking oral retinoids for acne, but is on no other medication. Except for the rash clinical examination is normal, no organomegaly, no lymphadenopathy. The patient experiences some symptomatic relief from topical steroids, but a blood sample taken returns the following results:

Hb	131 g/l
MCV	89 fl
WCC	7.2 x 10^9/l
Differential: 55% neutrophils, 31% lymphocytes, 6% eosinophils	
Plt	210 x 10^9/l
ESR	16 mm/hr
Na	138 mmol/l
K	4.1 mmol/l
Urea	6.3 mmol/l
Albumin	30 g/l
Bilirubin	16 µmol/l
ALT	19 U/l

1. Which of the following tests is likely to be the most useful?

- ❑ A Endoscopy and small bowel biopsy
- ❑ B Skin biopsy
- ❑ C Stool microscopy and cultures
- ❑ D Small bowel aspirate and culture
- ❑ E Small bowel enema

2. What is the likely diagnosis?

- ❑ A Whipple's disease
- ❑ B Cryptosporidium infection
- ❑ C Tropical sprue
- ❑ D Small bowel lymphoma
- ❑ E Coeliac disease

With the appropriate treatment the patient becomes asymptomatic, but presents two years later with prolonged episodes of diarrhoea.

3. What is the likely precipitating cause?

- ❑ A Malignant change
- ❑ B Bacterial overgrowth
- ❑ C Poor diet
- ❑ D Pseudomembranous colitis
- ❑ E Ileocaecal abscess

16 years later he is admitted as an emergency. The GP indicates that the patient has been asymptomatic up until the last six weeks when he started to lose weight and developed intermittent abdominal pain. On admission the patient is pale and has symptoms of small bowel obstruction.

4. What complication is likely to have developed?

- ❑ A Adhesions
- ❑ B Small bowel carcinoma
- ❑ C Ileo-caecal abscess
- ❑ D Small bowel lymphoma
- ❑ E Carcinoma of the colon

Case History 4 (9 marks)

A 63-year-old woman with an 18 year history of relapsing ulcerative colitis is admitted with increasing malaise and jaundice. She has lost 2 kg in weight over the last two months and was started on 30 mg prednisolone by her GP for worsening diarrhoea, three weeks ago. On examination, she looks unwell, there is scleral icterus and she is mildly dehydrated. Scratch marks are present over her arms and legs, there is no adenopathy, but a tender liver is palpable under the costal margins. The chest is clear and the examination of the CNS is unremarkable.

Hb	102 g/l
WCC	4.2 x 10^9/l
Plt	168 x 10^9/l
ESR	23 mm/hr
Na	131 mmol/l
K	3.9 mmol/l
Urea	4.2 mmol/l
Bilirubin	62 µmol/l
ALT	28 U/l
AST	35 U/l
Albumin	32 g/l

1. **What is the likely cause for her jaundice?**
2. **What test would you perform in the first instance?**

The patient has a biliary drain inserted and percutaneous cholangiogram shows irregular intrahepatic bile ducts, with a long, smooth stricture in the common hepatic duct and normal common bowel duct.

3. **What other differential diagnosis has to be considered?**
4. **What test would be the most useful at this stage?**

Case History 5 (8 marks)

A 29-year-old woman is admitted to the A&E Department with a severe episode of abdominal pain. In the past year she had three similar admissions to different hospitals, but was discharged after a few days with no specific diagnosis made. She was well until 15 months ago when she took an overdose of paracetamol and was started on fluoxetine by her GP. She is currently on no other medication. On examination she appears in pain. The abdomen is tender with some rebound pain and voluntary guarding. Bowel sounds are active. There is no hepato-splenomegaly or lymphadenopathy. Chest is clear. There is no focal neurology. Heart rate 104 sinus rhythm. BP 105/60 mmHg.

Hb	128 g/l
WCC	5.6 x 10^9/l
Plt	322 x 10^9/l
ESR	7 mm/hr
Na	128 mmol/l
K	3.5 mmol/l
Urea	4.0 mmol/l
BM	5 mmol/l
Dipstix Urine:	Protein ++, Blood -, Bilirubin +
Urine Osmolality	895 mosm/kg

1. **Suggest two investigations.**
2. **What is the likely diagnosis?**

The patient recovers spontaneously over the following two days.

3. **Give an important step in the further management.**

Case History 6 (10 marks)

A 24-year-old man is admitted to hospital with right loin pain. He was diagnosed as suffering from severe Haemophilia A at the age of three. His brother is also affected. He has advanced secondary degenerative changes of his knees, elbows and hips, but there is no other significant past medical history. On examination he is extremely tender in the right flank and has an extension deficit in the right hip of 20°. No haematoma is evident on inspection. There is some guarding in the right iliac fossa, bowel sounds are present. No organomegaly. Pulse rate 96/min, regular. BP 100/50 mmHg. An ejection systolic murmur is heard in the aortic region.

Hb	118 g/l
MCV	76 fl
WCC	8.2 x 10^9/l (63% neutrophils)
Plt	236 x 10^9/l
Electrolytes	Normal
Bilirubin	20 µmol/l
ALT	640 U/l
Albumin	34 g/l
INR	1.8
APTT	68 seconds
Dipstix Urine	Blood ++, Protein +, Ketones -

1. **What is the mode of inheritance?**
2. **What is the likely cause for the patient's presentation?**
3. **What is the likely underlying cause for the deranged liver function?**
4. **Suggest two investigations to confirm this.**

Case History 7 (10 marks)

A 19-year-old Indian man is admitted after two days of profound watery diarrhoea and colicky abdominal pain. He was previously perfectly well with normal developmental milestones. His elder brother who returned from a trip to Bangladesh three weeks previously has developed similar symptoms, although to a lesser degree.

On examination the patient is pyrexial 38.6 °C, he looks profoundly ill and is badly dehydrated. The abdomen is tender but soft. The bowel sounds are hyperactive. Liver and spleen are not enlarged and the chest is clear. Examination of the CNS is unremarkable.

Hb	159 g/l
WCC	7.8 x 10^9/l (normal differential)
Plt	361 x 10^9/l
Na	134 mmol/l
K	3.8 mmol/l
Urea	15.2 mmol/l
Creatinine	101 μmol/l

On the ward the patient has an episode of explosive diarrhoea, dipstix shows a trace of blood.

1. What test is most likely to be diagnostic?

- ❑ A Anal swab and microscopy
- ❑ B Stool microscopy and culture
- ❑ C Colonoscopy and full thickness biopsy
- ❑ D Serology for rotavirus
- ❑ E Small bowel aspirate and culture

After two days of aggressive resuscitation, the patient starts to recover, but on the third day after admission, develops tender erythematous lesions on both forearms. By this stage his brother has fully recovered and no other family member has become ill.

2. What complication is likely to have developed?

- ❑ A Erythema multiforme
- ❑ B Haemolytic uraemic syndrome
- ❑ C Henoch-Schönlein purpura
- ❑ D Bacterial endocarditis
- ❑ E Erythema nodosum

Over the following weeks the patient develops tender swellings of both wrists, the right shoulder and the left ankle. He also describes a very acute pain above his right buttock. He has sore eyes, a low grade pyrexia and mild shortness of breath.

3. What further test is likely to be the most useful?

- ❑ A X-ray of both wrists and pelvis
- ❑ B Chest X-ray
- ❑ C Joint aspiration and culture
- ❑ D Blood culture
- ❑ E Rheumatoid factor

4. What condition is likely to have developed?

- ❑ A Reactive arthritis
- ❑ B Bacterial endocarditis
- ❑ C Reiter's syndrome
- ❑ D Septic arthritis
- ❑ E Auto-immune vasculitis

5. What is the treatment?

- ❑ A Non-steroidal anti-inflammatory drugs
- ❑ B Six weeks of appropriate antibiotics
- ❑ C Reducing course of oral steroids
- ❑ D Low-dose Methotrexate
- ❑ E Intravenous immunoglobulins

Case History 8 (10 marks)

A 48-year-old stone mason is referred to clinic for investigation of a six-month history of malaise and weight gain. He is a non-smoking bachelor without a significant past medical history and is on no current medication. He admits to drinking half a bottle of spirits a day. On examination he has a healthy tan, is slightly overweight with normal conjunctivae and mucous membranes. The liver edge is palpable 3 cm under the costal margin. The spleen is not enlarged and there is no adenopathy. Examination of the chest and cardiovascular system is unremarkable. Examination of the legs shows mildly swollen and tender knees and reduction of light touch around the forefeet.

Full blood count	Normal
ESR	3 mm/hr
Na	139 mmol/l
K	4.1 mmol/l
Creatinine	108 μmol/l
ALT	98 U/l
Bilirubin	28 μmol/l

X-rays of the knees show advanced degenerative changes.

1. **Suggest two further investigations.**
2. **What is the likely underlying diagnosis?**
3. **How is it confirmed?**
4. **How is it acquired?**

Nine years later the patient is readmitted with a weight loss of 3 kg over the space of four months. The liver can no longer be palpated, but there is a smooth mass in the left upper quadrant.

Hb	187 g/l
PCV	66%
WCC	5.3 x 10^9/l
Plt	128 x 10^9/l
ESR	1 mm/hr
Normal U&E's	

5. **What important complication has to be excluded?**

GASTROENTEROLOGY QUESTIONS: DATA INTERPRETATIONS

For 'best-of-five' questions candidates must select one answer only, by putting a cross in the appropriate box.

Data Interpretation 1 (5 marks)

A 56-year-old veterinary is under investigation for recurrent chest and upper respiratory tract infections. He also gives a history of episodic diarrhoea over the last 18 months. Clinical examination is normal. His blood results show:

Full blood count	Normal
Electrolytes	Normal
Total protein	59 g/l
Albumin	51 g/l
IgG	4.5 g/l (normal 7.5–15)
IgA	0.3 g/l (normal 1.2–4.0)
IgM	0.3 g/l (normal 0.5–1.5)

1. What is the likely diagnosis?

❑ A Hodgkin disease
❑ B Non-Hodgkin's lymphoma
❑ C Acquired hypogammaglobinaemia
❑ D Kartagener's syndrome
❑ E Yellow nail syndrome

2. What is the most likely cause for the diarrhoea?

❑ A Villous atrophy
❑ B Maldigestion
❑ C Lymphoma of terminal ileum
❑ D Chronic giardia infection
❑ E Steatorrhoea

Data Interpretation 2 (6 marks)

A 19-year-old blood donor has the following blood results:

Bilirubin	36 μmol/l
Alkaline phosphatase	96 U/l
ALT	28 U/l
Haptoglobin	78 mg/dl (40–220 mg/dl)
Dipstix urine	Normal

1. What is the likely diagnosis?

- ❑ A Hereditary spherocytosis
- ❑ B Dubin-Johnson syndrome
- ❑ C Gilbert's syndrome
- ❑ D Rotor syndrome
- ❑ E Budd-Chiari syndrome

2. How is the condition transmitted?

- ❑ A Autosomal dominant
- ❑ B Autosomal recessive
- ❑ C X-linked dominant
- ❑ D X-linked recessive
- ❑ E Sporadic

3. What test is confirmatory?

- ❑ A Liver biopsy
- ❑ B Auto-antibody profile
- ❑ C Red cell membrane electrophoresis
- ❑ D Hepatic angiogram
- ❑ E Nicotinic acid test

Data Interpretation 3 (4 marks)

A 49-year-old woman complains of difficulty swallowing, recurrent episodes of sore eyes and generalised itch. She is not jaundiced, but she has periorbital xanthelasmata. The following results are obtained:

Hb	118 g/l
WCC	3.2 x 10^9/l
Plt	281 x 10^9/l
ESR	28 mm/hr
Albumin	36 g/l
Total protein	88 g/l
3 day faecal fat excretion	42 g

1. Which of the following tests would be the most useful?

- ❑ A Liver function test
- ❑ B Hepatitis serology
- ❑ C Protein electrophoresis
- ❑ D Antibodies to double stranded DNA
- ❑ E Anti-mitochondrial antibodies

2. What is the likely diagnosis?

- ❑ A Chronic persistent hepatitis
- ❑ B Chronic aggressive hepatitis
- ❑ C Primary biliary cirrhosis
- ❑ D Sclerosing cholangitis
- ❑ E Mixed connective tissue syndrome

Data Interpretation 4 (4 marks)

A 42-year-old vagrant is admitted to the A&E Department, with the following results:

Hb	109 g/l
MCV	101 g/l
WCC	4.8 x 10^9/l
Plt	197 x 10^9/l
Blood film	rouleaux formation, reticulocytes 5%
Na	108 mmol/l
K	5.6 mmol/l
Urea	2.8 mmol/l
Total cholesterol	9.6 mmol/l
Bilirubin	48 μmol/l
Direct Bilirubin	16 μmol/l (normal <5 μmol/l)

1. What is the diagnosis?

- ❑ A Acute alcoholic hepatitis
- ❑ B Zieve syndrome
- ❑ C Rhabdomyolysis
- ❑ D Scurvy
- ❑ E Methanol intoxication

2. What is the cause for the hyponatraemia?

- ❑ A Inappropriate ADH-secretion
- ❑ B Hyper-aldosteronism
- ❑ C Water intoxication
- ❑ D Central diabetes insipidus
- ❑ E Spurious hyponatraemia

Data Interpretation 5 (6 marks)

A 26-year-old woman is under investigation at the infertility clinic for malaise and secondary amenorrhoea. On examination she is moderately obese with abdominal striae and spider naevi. A firm tender liver edge can just be palpated under the right costal margin. Investigations show:

Hb	113 g/l
WBC	4.8 x 10^9/l
Plt	128 x 10^9/l
Electrolytes	Normal
Albumin	32 g/l
Total protein	86 g/l
Bilirubin	92 µmol/l
AST	512 U/l

1. What is the most likely diagnosis?

- ❑ A Haemochromatosis
- ❑ B Autoimmune chronic active hepatitis
- ❑ C Wilson's disease
- ❑ D Alpha-1 antitrypsin deficiency
- ❑ E Hepatitis E

2. Which of the following is the most important investigation?

- ❑ A Liver ultrasound
- ❑ B ERCP
- ❑ C Hepatitis serology
- ❑ D Coeruloplasmin level
- ❑ E Liver biopsy

3. What treatment would you recommend?

- ❑ A Azathioprine
- ❑ B Immunoglobulins
- ❑ C Liver transplant
- ❑ D Repeated venesection
- ❑ E D-penicillamine

Data Interpretation 6 (6 marks)

A 56-year-old man gives a four month history of abdominal pain, diarrhoea and weight loss of 2 kg. He had a partial gastrectomy at the age of 40. The following results are obtained:

Full blood count	Normal
Bilirubin	20 μmol/l
Albumin	34 g/l
ALT	59 U/l
3 day faecal fat excretion	18g per day/54g total

Urinary xylose excretion after 25 g oral D-xylose:
8g/5 hrs (normal > 6g/5 hrs)

1. **What is the most likely diagnosis?**
2. **What are the two most likely underlying causes?**
3. **Suggest two further tests.**

Data Interpretation 7 (4 marks)

A 63-year-old man is referred for an investigation of episodic bloating and diarrhoea. He was treated in his forties for presumed recurrent duodenal ulcers. The following results are obtained:

Hb	104 g/l
MCV	103 fl
WCC	6.2×10^9/l
Plt	217×10^9/l
Electrolytes	Normal

1. Suggest a diagnosis for the patient's symptoms.

An oral glucose tolerance test shows:

Time (mins)	Plasma glucose [mmol/l]
0	4.5
30	10.1
60	6.3
120	4.8

2. Suggest a further investigation.

Data Interpretation 8 (5 marks)

A 54-year-old man presents with a 3-month history of polyarthralgia and mild pyrexia up to 37.8 °C. Over the last month he has developed a diarrhoea which intermittently he has found difficult to flush down the toilet. The following results are obtained

Hb	114 g/l
MCV	98 fl
WCC	5.6 x 10^9/l (normal differential)
Plt	322 x 10^9/l
Total protein	60 g/l
Globulin	35 g/l

A small bowel biopsy shows infiltration with PAS positive macrophages.

1. What is the likely diagnosis?

- ❑ A Non-Hodgkin's lymphoma
- ❑ B Small bowel tuberculosis
- ❑ C Whipple's disease
- ❑ D Panarteritis nodosa
- ❑ E Familial Mediterranean fever

2. How could the diagnosis be confirmed?

- ❑ A Lymph node biopsy
- ❑ B Stool culture
- ❑ C Joint aspiration for microscopy and culture
- ❑ D Polymerase chain reaction from duodenal biopsy
- ❑ E Autoantibody screen

Data Interpretation 9 (6 marks)

A 16-year-old boy is admitted after an episode of haematemesis. The only past history of note is a premature delivery at 30 weeks followed by hyaline membrane disease. The spleen is enlarged, the liver is not palpable. Gastroscopy shows oesophageal varices which are successfully injected and sclerosed. Ascites is found which shows the following biochemistry:

Specific gravity	1025
Protein	28 g/l
Glucose	5.8 mmol/l
Blood glucose	6.2 mmol/l

1. What do these results suggest?

- ❑ A Septic peritonitis
- ❑ B Portal vein thrombosis
- ❑ C Tuberculous peritonitis
- ❑ D End-stage liver cirrhosis
- ❑ E Budd-Chiari syndrome

2. What is the likely underlying cause?

- ❑ A Prolonged severe illness in the neonatal period
- ❑ B Umbilical vein catheterization
- ❑ C Hepatitis C following transfusion
- ❑ D Hypogammaglobulinaemia
- ❑ E Alpha-1 antitrypsin deficiency

After two days the patient has a further episode of haematemesis

3. What is the likely cause?

- ❑ A Mucosal necrosis following sclerotherapy
- ❑ B Boerhaave syndrome
- ❑ C Fundal varices
- ❑ D Recanalisation on the oesophageal varices
- ❑ E Acute on chronic liver failure due to GI haemorrhage

Data Interpretation 10 (5 marks)

A 23-year-old woman who is 33 weeks pregnant is referred to clinic for investigation of hypertension and proteinuria. Investigations show

Hb	99 g/l
WCC	6.4 x 10^9/l
Plt	58 x 10^9/l
Blood film	spherocytes and 'bite cells'
Bilirubin	196 μmol/l
ALT	350 mmol/l
Total protein	68 g/l
Urinalysis	Blood ++, Urobilinogen ++, Protein +++
INR	1.0

1. What is the diagnosis based on these results?

❑ A HELLP syndrome
❑ B Rhesus incompatibility
❑ C Acute fatty liver of pregnancy
❑ D Cholestasis of pregnancy
❑ E Eclampsia

2. What is the treatment?

❑ A Anti-Rhesus immunoglobulins
❑ B High-dose methylprednisolone
❑ C Exchange transfusion
❑ D Beta blockers
❑ E Delivery of baby

Data Interpretation 11 (6 marks)

A 52-year-old patient with an 18 year history of recurrent peptic ulcer disease is investigated for a further relapse. He has not undergone any previous surgery. These are the results of his secretin test:

Baseline gastrin	380 pmol/l
After injection of secretin (2U/kg)	280 pmol/l (20–100 pmol/l)

1. **What is the most likely cause for these results?**
2. **Give two further differential diagnoses.**
3. **What is the next investigation?**

Data Interpretation 12 (5 marks)

A 56-year-old farmer is admitted with a sudden onset of right upper quadrant pain and mild jaundice. He has previously been well, but is now wheezy with a respiratory rate of 28 and a temperature of 38.7 °C. He has a blood pressure of 100/45 mmHg, pulse rate 112/min and a tender lobulated mass is palpable in the right flank.

Hb	141 g/l
MCV	88 fl
WCC	7.9 x 10^9/l
Differential: 64% neutrophils, 25% lymphocytes, 8% eosinophils	
Electrolytes	Normal
Dipstix Urine	Blood -, Protein -, Bilirubin ++

6 hours later the patient has a generalised seizure.

1. What is the likely diagnosis?

❑ A Adult polycystic disease
❑ B Tuberous sclerosis
❑ C Liver abscesses
❑ D Wegener's granulomatosis
❑ E Hydatid disease

2. What is the next investigation?

❑ A CT abdomen
❑ B Chest X-ray
❑ C EEG
❑ D Blood cultures
❑ E CT brain

Data Interpretation 13 (5 marks)

A 42-year-old woman is admitted for investigation of nocturnal fits. Her weight has increased by 3 kg over the last six months. Three separate early morning glucose samples were obtained with the following results:

Monday	4.6 mmol/l
Tuesday	2.3 mmol/l
Wednesday	7.8 mmol/l

C-peptide after 24 hour fast 1.8 nmol/l (normal 0.2–0.6 nmol/l)

1. What diagnosis do these results suggest?

❑ A Glucagonoma
❑ B Self-administration of insulin
❑ C Multiple Endocrine Neoplasia Type II
❑ D Insulinoma
❑ E Maturity onset of diabetes in the young (MODY)

2. What is the next investigation?

❑ A Repeat C-peptide after 72 hour fast
❑ B Estimation of pro-insulin
❑ C Oral glucose tolerance test
❑ D CT pancreas
❑ E Insulin stress test

Data Interpretation 14 (5 marks)

A 71-year-old woman is investigated for the following results:

Hb	94 g/l
MCV	71 fl
WCC	4.8×10^9/l
Plt	134×10^9/l
ESR	52 mm/hr
Normal electrolytes	

She had a previous partial gastrectomy three years ago for a 'growth'. Clinical examination demonstrates ascites. On aspiration clear, gelatinous fluid is obtained. A chest X-ray shows right hilar adenopathy and pleural effusion.

1. How do you explain the appearance of the ascites?

- ❑ A Tuberculous peritonitis
- ❑ B Pseudomyxoma peritonei
- ❑ C Aspiration of giant ovarian cyst
- ❑ D Aspiration of porcelain gall bladder
- ❑ E Diffuse lymphoma

2. What is the likely diagnosis?

- ❑ A Disseminated tuberculosis
- ❑ B Ovarian teratodermoid
- ❑ C Peritoneal mesothelioma
- ❑ D Krukenberg metastases
- ❑ E Non-Hodgkin's lymphoma

Data Interpretation 15 (6 marks)

A 69-year-old diabetic is admitted with right upper quadrant pain, and rigors. His bowel habit has been irregular for the last three years and has had intermittent left iliac fossa pain. His investigations show

Hb	98 g/l
MCV	82 fl
WCC	9.1 x 10^9/l
Differential: 85% neutrophils, 12% lymphocytes	
Plt	512 x 10^9/l
ESR	78 mm/hr
Electrolytes	Normal
Bilirubin	22 µmol/l
ALT	56 U/l
Albumin	22 g/l
Total protein	71 g/l

1. What investigation is likely to be the most useful?

- ❑ A Blood cultures
- ❑ B Abdominal ultrasound
- ❑ C Barium enema
- ❑ D Radionucleide white cell scan
- ❑ E Chest X-ray

2. What is the likely underlying cause?

- ❑ A Streptococcal liver abscess
- ❑ B Mycobacterial empyema
- ❑ C Emphysematous cholecystitis
- ❑ D Enterococcal peri-nephric abscess
- ❑ E *E. coli* psoas abscess

3. What treatment would you recommend

- ❑ A Oral co-amoxiclav
- ❑ B Intravenous erythromycin
- ❑ C Oral anti-tuberculous triple therapy
- ❑ D iv benzyl-penicillin plus gentamicin
- ❑ E Percutaneous drainage

Data Interpretation 16 (6 marks)

A 17-year-old girl is investigated for a Parkinsonian syndrome. This has insidiously presented over the space of two years with a low frequency tremor, rigor in the upper limbs and a dysarthria. The following are the results of a glucose tolerance test after 75 grams of oral disaccharides:

Time	Glucose [mmol/l]
0	4.6
30	12.8
60	10.9
90	6.5
120	3.2

1. **What abnormality is shown?**
2. **What is the likely diagnosis?**
3. **How would you confirm it?**

HAEMATOLOGY QUESTIONS: CASE HISTORIES

For 'best-of-five' questions candidates must select one answer only, by putting a cross in the appropriate box.

Case History 1 (9 marks)

A 59-year-old female is being referred for investigation of amaurosis fugax. She has been started on enalapril and low-dose aspirin six-months previously by her GP for newly diagnosed hypertension and one TIA affecting her left arm.

She has been previously well, smokes 15 cigarettes per day and drinks two glasses of sherry per night.

On examination she looks extremely well. BP 165/95 mmHg, pulse 68/min regular, on auscultation 2/6 ejection systolic murmur over the aorta.

The lungs are clear. A mass is palpable in the left upper quadrant, no enlarged lymph nodes are found. Examination of the CNS is unremarkable.

The following blood results are obtained:

Hb	158 g/l
MCV	67 fl
MCHC	26 g/dl
WCC	14.2 x 10^9/l
Differential: neutrophils 83%, lymphocytes 11%, monocytes 5%	
Plt	489 x 10^9/l
PCV	0.58
Blood film	Hypochromia, polychromasia
Biochemical profile	Normal

1. What examination is least likely to be useful?

- ❑ A Chest X-ray
- ❑ B Erythrocyte sedimentation rate
- ❑ C Ultrasound abdomen
- ❑ D Arterial blood gases
- ❑ E Bone marrow biopsy

While on the ward, the patient has a severe episode of epistaxis.

2. Which of the following tests is likely to be normal?

❑ A Bleeding time
❑ B Uric acid levels
❑ C Free iron binding capacity
❑ D Erythropoietin
❑ E Prothrombin time

3. What is the treatment?

❑ A 5-hydroxyurea
❑ B Aspirin
❑ C Venaesection
❑ D Methotrexate
❑ E Splenectomy

The patient is treated successfully and makes a good recovery. Seven years later, however, she is re-admitted with the following results:

Hb 91 g/l
WCC 2.8 x 10^9/l
Plt 93 x 10^9/l
Blood film: Multiple nucleated red cells, myeloblasts and megakaryocytes
ESR 52 mm/hr

On examination, the patient is pale and several ecchymoses are present over arms and trunk. A firm mass is occupying the whole of the abdomen.

4. What complication has arisen?

❑ A Chronic myeloid leukaemia
❑ B Aplastic anaemia
❑ C Iron depletion
❑ D Myelofibrosis
❑ E Acute myelo-monocytic leukaemia

Case History 2 (9 marks)

A 9-year-old foster child is brought into hospital extremely unwell. He is complaining of severe abdominal pain and is unable to lie still.

On examination the patient has a pyrexia of 38.9 °C. He is pale with a sinus tachycardia of 132/min. Respiratory rate is 40/min and the right lung base is dull on percussion with increased vocal resonance.

The abdomen is tender to palpation with peritonism, however rebound is negative and the bowel sounds are hyperactive but of normal quality. A blood sample taken in the resuscitation room yields the following results:

Hb	89 g/l
MCV	100 fl
WCC	14.1 x 10^9/l
Plt	439 x 10^9/l
Na	141 mmol/l
K	5.2 mmol/l
Urea	10.8 mmol/l
Creatinine	88 µmol/l
Dipstix urine	Blood ++, Protein -, Ketones -
Arterial blood gases (on air)	
pH	7.51
pO_2	8.6 kPa
pCO_2	3.8 kPa
HCO_3^-	21 mmol/l

An abdominal X-ray shows a normal bowel gas pattern but sclerotic areas within the pelvic bones.
A chest X-ray shows right lower lobe consolidation.

1. **Which combination of the following investigations would you request?**

- ❑ A White cell differential and bone marrow biopsy
- ❑ B Sputum culture and ultrasound abdomen
- ❑ C Blood cultures and standard blood film
- ❑ D Urine serology and blood clotting
- ❑ E Thick film microscopy and Gram stain of sputum

2. What immediate management would you advise?

- ❑ A Resuscitation and iv penicillin
- ❑ B iv morphine and iv doxycycline
- ❑ C Blood transfusion and iv hydrocortisone
- ❑ D High dose oxygen and iv gentamycin
- ❑ E Forced diuresis and iv heparin

Over the next two weeks, the patient makes a good recovery and is about to be discharged.

3. What further treatment is important?

- ❑ A Prolonged course of antibiotics
- ❑ B Pneumococcal vaccination
- ❑ C Prophylactic antibiotics
- ❑ D Monitoring of blood film
- ❑ E Monitoring of renal function

Two years later, the patient is re-admitted to hospital two weeks after a febrile illness. He is pale and short of breath at rest. There is evidence of a bilateral, asymmetrical arthropathy affecting the elbows, wrists and knees.

The following results are obtained:

Hb	42 g/l
MCV	91 fl
WCC	3.1×10^9/l
Plt	102×10^9/l

Blood film: Profound anaemia, numerous Howell-Jolly bodies, multiple hypersegmented neutrophils

4. What is the likely cause for these results?

- ❑ A Idiosyncratic drug reaction
- ❑ B Acute leukaemia
- ❑ C Drug toxicity
- ❑ D Secondary lymphoma
- ❑ E Viral infection

Case History 3 (9 marks)

A 59-year-old publican presents with two episodes of haematemesis in the space of 24 hours. He has a several month history of mild dyspepsia but has not required any specific treatment. Two years previously he had developed a full length thrombosis of his right leg, following a cholecystectomy. He was treated with warfarin for three months and had made a good recovery. On admission he is on no regular medication, but smokes 15 cigarettes per day and drinks two to three pints of beer daily.

On examination, he is pale, blood pressure 135/75 mmHg, pulse 92/min regular, no murmurs. Chest is clear. Abdominal examination reveals a spleen palpable 3 cm below the left costal margin, but no associated hepatomegaly. He is not jaundiced and no spider naevi can be found. PR examination reveals melaena stools but no palpable mass.

Investigations show the following results:

Hb	112 g/l
MCV	66 fl
WCC	14.6 x 10^9/l
Differential: 91% neutrophils, 6% lymphocytes, 2% monocytes	
Plt	917 x 10^9/l
MCH	24 pg
MCHC	30 g/dl

Na	139 mmol/l
K	4.9 mmol/l
Urea	17.2 mmol/l
Creatinine	127 µmol/l
Albumin	37 g/l
AST	52 U/l
Gamma-GT	197 U/l
Uric acid	536 µmol/l (< 420 µmol/l)

Gastroscopy shows a normal oesophagus but a bleeding pre-pyloric ulcer which is successfully injected with alcohol. Biopsy from the margin shows no malignant cells.

1. What examination would you perform next?

- ❑ A Philadelphia-chromosome
- ❑ B Alkaline leucocyte phosphatase (ALP)
- ❑ C Blood film
- ❑ D Repeat gastric biopsy
- ❑ E CT abdomen

2. What treatment would you recommend?

- ❑ A Aspirin
- ❑ B Intravenous heparin
- ❑ C Gastrectomy
- ❑ D Splenectomy
- ❑ E α-interferon

The following day the patient deteriorates and the following results are obtained:

Hb	109 g/l
WCC	13.6 x 10^9/l
Plt	871 x 10^9/l
Na	135 mmol/l
K	5.1 mmol/l
Urea	31 mmol/l
Creatinine	238 μmol/l
Dipstix urine	Blood +++, Protein +, Bilirubin -

3. What complication has occurred?

- ❑ A Obstructing renal stone
- ❑ B Renal vein thrombosis
- ❑ C Cerebral haemorrhage
- ❑ D Recurrent GI-haemorrhage
- ❑ E Acute hepatic failure

4. What is the underlying diagnosis?

- ❑ A Metastatic gastric carcinoma
- ❑ B Chronic myeloid leukaemia
- ❑ C Essential thrombocythaemia
- ❑ D Waldenström's macroglobulinaemia
- ❑ E Kaposi's sarcoma

Case History 4 (10 marks)

A 29-year-old female accountant presents with a swollen right leg. One year previously she had been on warfarin for a suspected pulmonary embolism, however she had refused VQ-lung scan as she thought she was pregnant at the time. She is otherwise well and on no regular medication except simple analgesics for tension headaches.

The following results are obtained:

Hb	106 g/l
MCV	103 fl
WCC	6.1 x 10^9/l (63% neutrophils)
RCC	2.9 x 10^{12}/l (7% reticulocytes)
Plt	172 x 10^9/l
PT	15 s (control 12–14 s)
APTT	78 s (control 32 s)
APTT after 1:1 addition of normal plasma	72 s
Bleeding time	6 min (5–8 min)
Na	136 mmol/l
K	5.1 mmol/l
Creatinine	151 μmol/l
Direct Coombs' test	Positive

1. What do the clotting results suggest?

- ❑ A Platelet defect
- ❑ B Defect in extrinsic clotting pathway
- ❑ C Defect in intrinsic clotting pathway
- ❑ D Anti-phospholipid antibodies
- ❑ E Red cell defect

2. What is the cause for the anaemia?

- ❑ A Chronic disease
- ❑ B Auto-immune haemolytic anaemia
- ❑ C Sideroblastic anaemia
- ❑ D Vitamin B_{12} deficiency
- ❑ E Hypersplenism

3. What is the next investigation?

- ❑ A Haemoglobin electrophoresis
- ❑ B Indirect Coombs' test
- ❑ C Ultrasound abdomen
- ❑ D Red cell sequestration studies
- ❑ E Auto-antibody screen

Ten months later, the patient presents to the eye hospital complaining of a 'dark cloud' in the top right corner of her right eye. Fundoscopy shows a focal haemorrhage in the right retina, the remainder of the retina and the left fundus are normal. Her blood pressure is found to be 155/100 mmHg and a trace of protein is found in the urine.

4. What is the likely cause for the visual problem?

- ❑ A Retinal vein branch occlusion
- ❑ B Retinal artery branch occlusion
- ❑ C Hypertensive haemorrhage
- ❑ D Retinal detachment
- ❑ E Amaurosis fugax

5. What treatment would you recommend?

- ❑ A Heparin
- ❑ B Aspirin
- ❑ C Warfarin
- ❑ D Fresh frozen plasma
- ❑ E Laser treatment

Case History 5 (7 marks)

A 10-year-old boy is under investigation for suspected bilateral Perthes' disease of the hip. While on bed rest, awaiting investigation, he develops painful swelling of the right leg.

Examination of the abdomen shows no enlargement of liver or spleen, and there is no adenopathy. The chest is clear. The circumference of the mid-thigh on the right is increased by 2 cm when compared with the left. No cellulitis is seen.

The following results are obtained:

Hb	142 g/l
WCC	6.7 x 10^9/l
Plt	338 x 10^9/l
ESR	31mm/hr
Biochemical profile	Normal
PT	12 s (control 12–14 s)
APTT	31 s (control 32–34 s)
Bleeding time	5.5 min (5–8 min)
D-dimer	960 μg/l (20–400 μg/l)

1. Which of the following examinations is likely to be least useful?

- ❑ A Thrombin time
- ❑ B Doppler-Ultrasound
- ❑ C Protein C levels
- ❑ D Protein S levels
- ❑ E Anti-thrombin levels

The patient is fully anti-coagulated with low-molecular heparin. Two days later, whilst still on bed rest, he develops a tender swelling of the left calf. A venogram is performed which demonstrates thrombosis of two pairs of calf veins but patent popliteal and femoral veins.

2. What is the most likely diagnosis?

- ❑ A Protein C deficiency
- ❑ B Protein S deficiency
- ❑ C Disseminated intravascular coagulation
- ❑ D Anti-thrombin III deficiency
- ❑ E Haemoglobin C disease

An ultrasound scan of the abdomen and a chest X-ray are normal. While awaiting the results of further investigations, oral anti-coagulants are withheld. One week later the patient develops bruising over the extensor surfaces and has a severe episode of epistaxis.

The following results are obtained:

Hb	138 g/l
WCC	6.2×10^9/l
Plt	32×10^9/l
Prothrombin time	13 s (control 12–14 s)

3. What is the likely cause for the haemorrhage?

❑ A Disseminated intravascular coagulation
❑ B Heparin overdose
❑ C Hypersplenism
❑ D Heparin side-effect
❑ E Factor VIII depletion

Case History 6 (9 marks)

A 53-year-old widower is referred from his GP because of easy bruising and malaise. He has recently had recurrent upper respiratory tract infections but is otherwise well.

He takes ibuprofen for arthritis and peppermint oil for irritable bowel syndrome. On examination he is pale, no palpable organomegaly, no lymphadenopathy. Examination of chest and cardiovascular system is unremarkable.

The following results are obtained:

Hb	98 g/l
MCV	81 fl
WCC	4.1 x 10^9/l
Plt	108 x 10^9/l
ESR	53 mm/hr

Blood film: Target cells, < 0.5% reticulocytes, 2% blasts, occasional ring sideroblast

Na	136 mmol/l
K	3.8 mmol/l
Creatinine	136 μmol/l
Albumin	41 g/l
Total protein	75 g/l
Liver function tests	Normal
Chest X-ray	Normal

1. **Suggest one further investigation.**
2. **What is the likely diagnosis?**

The patient is treated supportively only requiring the occasional blood transfusion, but 18 months later is admitted with a cough and shortness of breath. His full blood count shows:

Hb	69 g/l
WCC	8.9 x 10^9/l
Plt	83 x 10^9/l
Blood film	12% blasts, multiple Auer rods

Chest X-ray shows a small area of consolidation in right upper lobe with central cavitation. No pleural effusion, no adenopathy.

3. **What is the likely cause for the respiratory symptoms?**
4. **What do the blood results suggest?**

Case History 7 (7 marks)

A 72-year-old farmer complains of progressive shortness of breath and increasing fatigue. He recently required a course of antibiotics from his GP for a chest infection. He complains of occasional indigestion and, on two occasions, has noticed some dark blood in his stools. There is no history of haematuria, haemoptysis or bruising. His health is otherwise good with a steady weight and good appetite. He is an ex-smoker and drinks approximately two units of alcohol per night. His only other complaint is of long-standing lower backache.

On examination he is pale, no lymphadenopathy, BP 140/80 mmHg, chest clear, abdominal examination unremarkable.
Investigations show:

Hb	86 g/l
MCV	70 fl
WCC	9.5 x 10^9/l
Plt	479 x 10^9/l
MCH	17.1 pg
MCHC	22.9 g/dl
Haematocrit	38%

Blood film: Microcyctic, hypochromic, some rouleaux formation

Na	138 mmol/l
K	4.6 mmol/l
Urea	7.9 mmol/l
Creatinine	136 µmol/l
Calcium	2.15 mmol/l
Albumin	38 g/l
Total protein	95 g/l
Alkaline phosphatase	95 U/l
Serum electrophoresis	Narrow peak in the gamma region

Lumbar spine X-ray	Old wedge fracture of L1
Bone marrow biopsy	6% plasma cells
Barium enema	Normal

Mesenteric angiography shows an abnormal vascular blush in the ascending colon

1. What is the likely cause for the anaemia?

- ❑ A Colonic carcinoma
- ❑ B Colonic varices
- ❑ C Angiodysplasia
- ❑ D Meckel's diverticulum
- ❑ E Caecal lymphoma

2. What therapy would you recommend?

- ❑ A Right hemicolectomy
- ❑ B Resection of terminal ileum
- ❑ C Chemotherapy
- ❑ D Porto-caval shunt
- ❑ E Endoscopic sclerotherapy

3. How do you interpret the immune electrophoresis?

- ❑ A Reactive elevation
- ❑ B Myeloma
- ❑ C Waldenström's macroglobulinaemia
- ❑ D Benign monoclonal gammopathy
- ❑ E Lymphoma

HAEMATOLOGY QUESTIONS: DATA INTERPRETATIONS

For 'best-of-five' questions candidates must select one answer only, by putting a cross in the appropriate box.

Data Interpretation 1 (6 marks)

A 21-year-old woman is brought to the Accident & Emergency Department by her mother with a three-day history of fevers to 39 °C with associated rigors and increasing confusion.

The blood results show:

Hb	89 g/l
MCV	76 fl
RCC	2.6×10^{12}/l (0.2% reticulocytes)
WCC	1.1×10^{9}/l (95% lymphocytes, no blasts)
Plt	23×10^{9}/l

1. What investigation would you perform?

❑ A EBV antibody titres
❑ B Throat swab
❑ C Bone marrow biopsy
❑ D Lumbar puncture
❑ E Serum and urine drug screen

2. Which of the following diagnoses is least likely?

❑ A Acute myeloid leukaemia
❑ B Hodgkin disease
❑ C Drug induced aplastic anaemia
❑ D Post-viral aplastic anaemia
❑ E Idiopathic aplastic anaemia

3. What is the immediate management?

❑ A iv immunoglobulins
❑ B Transfusion of granulocytes
❑ C Stimulators of granulopoiesis (GM-CSF)
❑ D iv antibiotics
❑ E iv hydrocortisone

Data Interpretation 2 (6 marks)

A 7-year-old boy suffers excessive haemorrhage during appendicectomy. His mother has noticed small petechial skin haemorrhage in the past. Investigations show:

Hb	119 g/l
WCC	7.9 x 10^9/l, normal differential
Plt	357 x 10^9/l
Blood film: Normal except for mild reticulocytosis of 3%	
PT	14 s (control 12–14 s)
APTT	35 s (control 31–33 s)
Factor VIII activity	79%
Factor IX	99%

1. What further investigation would you perform?

- ❑ A Bleeding time
- ❑ B Thrombin time
- ❑ C Platelet antibodies
- ❑ D Red cell sequestration studies
- ❑ E Factor XI activity

2. What therapy would you recommend?

- ❑ A Plasmapheresis
- ❑ B Oral prednisolone
- ❑ C Splenectomy
- ❑ D Symptomatic therapy only
- ❑ E Dipyridamole

3. What is the aetiology of the condition?

- ❑ A Idiopathic
- ❑ B Post-infectious
- ❑ C X-linked recessive
- ❑ D Autosomal dominant
- ❑ E Autosomal recessive

Data Interpretation 3 (6 marks)

A 28-year-old Ghanaian woman attends the antenatal clinic with her first pregnancy. Her last menstrual period was normal seven weeks previously.

The following results are obtained:

Hb	109 g/l
MCV	86 fl
WCC	6.2 x 10^9/l
Plt	238 x 10^9/l
Haemoglobin electrophoresis	HbA 61% (HbA_2 5.5%), HbS 39%

Her partner is screened and the following results are found:

Hb	116 g/l
RCC	5.9 x 10^{12}/l
MCV	65 fl
Haemoglobin electrophoresis	HbA 84% (HbA_2 12%), HbF 16%

1. **What is the diagnosis in the mother?**
2. **What is the diagnosis in the father?**
3. **What is the likelihood of the child inheriting a severe haemoglobinopathy?**

Data Interpretation 4 (4 marks)

A 26-year-old woman has become profoundly unwell after Caesarean section for monozygotic twins.
Investigations show:

Hb	93 g/l
MCV	96 fl
WCC	10.2 x 10^9/l (87% neutrophils)
Plt	51 x 10^9/l
Blood film: Reticulocytosis, red cell fragmentation	
PT	21 s (control 12–14 s)
APTT	42 s (control 34 s)
Thrombin time	29 s (control 16 s)

1. Which of the two following tests would you perform?

- ❑ A Fibrin degradation products (FDP) and anti-thrombin levels
- ❑ B Thrombin time with protamine and chest X-ray
- ❑ C D-dimer levels and blood cultures
- ❑ D Abdominal ultrasound scan and bleeding time
- ❑ E Biochemical profile and arterial blood gases

2. What is the most likely underlying cause?

- ❑ A Pelvic sepsis
- ❑ B Amniotic fluid embolus
- ❑ C Ligation of iliac artery
- ❑ D Perforation of colon
- ❑ E Pyelonephritis

Data Interpretation 5 (4 marks)

A 37-year-old Hindu woman presents with tiredness and menorrhagia. The following results are obtained:

Hb	91 g/l
MCV	108 fl
WCC	3.1×10^9/l
Plt	128×10^9/l
Biochemical profile	Normal
Serum Gastrin	31 pmol/l (20–100 pmol/l)

1. **What is the most likely diagnosis?**
2. **Suggest two further investigations.**

Data Interpretation 6 (4 marks)

A 72-year-old woman is under investigation for back pain. It is noted that she passes 2.5 litres of urine per day.

A radio-isotope bone scan shows no abnormal areas of increased activity.

The following blood results are obtained:

Hb	94 g/l
WCC	4.1 x 10^9/l
Plt	128 x 10^9/l
MCV	85 fl
MCHC	31 g/dl
Blood film; Normocytic anaemia, rouleaux formation ++	
Urinary protein electrophoresis	Normal

1. What is the likely diagnosis?

- ❑ A Spinal tuberculosis
- ❑ B Chronic lymphocytic leukaemia
- ❑ C Multiple myeloma
- ❑ D Waldenström's macroglobulinaemia
- ❑ E Metastasised carcinoma of the breast

2. Which of the following tests is going to be least useful?

- ❑ A Biochemical profile
- ❑ B ESR
- ❑ C Chest X-ray
- ❑ D Serum protein electrophoresis
- ❑ E Bone marrow aspiration

Data Interpretation 7 (5 marks)

A 9-year-old boy is admitted with acute abdominal pain. On examination he is pale and of small stature.

A hand X-ray shows a skeletal maturity of approximately 4.5 years and dense bands across the metacarpal metaphyses.

Hb	101 g/l
MCV	81 fl
WCC	6.3 x 10^9/l
Plt	183 x 10^9/l
MCH	21 pg

Blood film: Di-morphic erythropoiesis, occasional ringsideroblast

1. What is the likely diagnosis?

- ❑ A Wilson's disease
- ❑ B Glue sniffing
- ❑ C Hereditary sideroblastic anaemia
- ❑ D Acute leukaemia
- ❑ E Lead poisoning

2. What simple tests may confirm the diagnosis?

- ❑ A Abdominal X-ray
- ❑ B Ham's test
- ❑ C Abdominal ultrasound
- ❑ D ESR
- ❑ E White cell differential

Data Interpretation 8 (5 marks)

A 76-year-old man is referred by his GP for episodes of acrocyanosis when washing his hands.
The fingers directly develop a purple discoloration after exposure to cold water. No blanching phase is observed.

Blood samples obtained in the evening show the following results:

Na	138 mmol/l
K	3.9 mmol/l
Urea	6.3 mmol/l
Creatinine	121 µmol/l
Albumin	39 g/l
Total protein	83 g/l

The full blood count sample is kept in the fridge overnight and the following day the pathology staff request a new sample as it has haemolysed.

1. Which of the following investigations is likely to be most helpful?

- ❑ A White cell differential
- ❑ B Blood film
- ❑ C Immune electrophoresis
- ❑ D Rheumatoid factor
- ❑ E Bone marrow biopsy

2. What is the likely diagnosis?

- ❑ A Chronic lymphocytic leukaemia
- ❑ B Paroxysmal nocturnal haemoglobinuria
- ❑ C Cold haemagglutinin disease
- ❑ D Hereditary spherocytosis
- ❑ E Mixed connective tissue disease

Data Interpretation 9 (4 marks)

A 28-year-old Asian man is investigated for night sweats and low-grade pyrexia. He has also developed an intolerance to alcohol. Clinical examination is normal. Blood samples show the following results:

Hb	132 g/l
WCC	4.7 x 10^9/l (87% neutrophils, 7% eosinophils)
Plt	218 x 10^9/l
ESR	56 mm/hr
Ultrasound abdomen	Normal

1. What is the likely diagnosis?

- ❑ A Pulmonary aspergillosis
- ❑ B Non-Hodgkin's lymphoma
- ❑ C Hodgkin disease
- ❑ D Hydatid disease
- ❑ E Pulmonary eosinophilia

2. Which of the following treatments would you recommend?

- ❑ A Radiotherapy
- ❑ B Chemotherapy
- ❑ C Amphoteracin B
- ❑ D Surgical excision
- ❑ E Oral prednisolone

Data Interpretation 10 (5 marks)

A 30-year-old Nigerian woman requires a four unit blood transfusion for post-partum haemorrhage after the birth of her second child.

Five days later she is noted to have scleral icterus and the following blood results are obtained:

Hb	83 g/l
MCV	101 fl
WCC	10.9 x 10^9/l (76% neutrophils)
Plt	604 x 10^9/l
Blood film	Di-morphic, 8% reticulocytes
Dipstix urine	Protein -, Blood +++, Glucose -

1. Which of the following tests would you perform?

- ❑ A Indirect Coombs' test
- ❑ B Direct Coombs' test
- ❑ C Osmotic resistance
- ❑ D Donath-Landsteiner test
- ❑ E Ham's test

2. What is the likely diagnosis?

- ❑ A Rhesus incompatibility between mother and child
- ❑ B ABO incompatibility between mother and child
- ❑ C Delayed transfusion reaction
- ❑ D Acquired auto-immune haemolysis
- ❑ E Post-partal sepsis

Data Interpretation 11 (4 marks)

A 54-year-old woman with long-standing active rheumatoid arthritis is referred for the investigation of anaemia. Her blood results show:

Hb	94 g/l
MCV	99 fl
WCC	4.2 x 10^9/l (76% neutrophils)
Plt	173 x 10^9/l
ESR	32 mm/hr

1. **Which of the following is unlikely to be the cause for these results?**

- ❑ A Methotrexate
- ❑ B Sulphasalazine
- ❑ C Gold
- ❑ D Hypothyroidism
- ❑ E Pernicious anaemia

2. **Which of the following tests would be the most helpful?**

- ❑ A B_{12}-levels
- ❑ B Folate levels
- ❑ C Haptoglobin levels
- ❑ D Blood film
- ❑ E Gastroscopy and biopsy

Data Interpretation 12 (2 marks)

The following blood results are returned for a man on out-patient follow-up for recurrent episodes of ventricular tachycardia. His current medication is aspirin and amiodarone.

Na	131 mmol/l
K	7.1 mmol/l
Urea	19.2 mmol/l
Glucose	1.1 mmol/l

1. What would you expect to see in the blood film?

- ❑ A Normal appearances
- ❑ B Haemolysis
- ❑ C Basophilic stippling
- ❑ D Heinz bodies
- ❑ E Howell-Jolly bodies

Data Interpretation 13 (6 marks)

A 16-year-old Israeli boy is returned to the UK by air ambulance from a holiday in Kenya. He had not felt particularly ill, but on the second day he developed jaundice and frank haematuria. His pulse rate is 100/min, regular, BP 110/60 mmHg. His blood results show:

Hb	87 g/l
MCV	101 fl
WCC	5.9 x 10^9/l
Plt	329 x 10^9/l
ESR	34 mm/hr
Haptoglobin	12 mg/dl (50–200 mg/dl)

Blood film: Bite cells, extensive Heinz body formation, 11% reticulocytes

1. What is the most important step in the management?

- ❑ A Intravenous hydrocortisone
- ❑ B Discontinue any medication
- ❑ C Administration of two units O rh-negative blood
- ❑ D Plasmapheresis
- ❑ E Continue malaria prophylaxis

2. What is the likely diagnosis?

- ❑ A Glucose-6-phosphate-dehydrogenase deficiency
- ❑ B Rotor syndrome
- ❑ C Hereditary spherocytosis
- ❑ D Haemoglobin C disease
- ❑ E Hereditary elliptocytosis

3. What is the inheritance of this condition?

- ❑ A Sporadic
- ❑ B Autosomal dominant
- ❑ C Autosomal recessive
- ❑ D X-linked dominant
- ❑ E X-linked recessive

Data Interpretation 14 (4 marks)

A 56-year-old labourer complains of headaches and episodes of dizziness. He is on bumetanide and smokes 40 cigarettes a day.

On examination he has evidence of chronic airways disease, blood pressure 170/95 mmHg. Investigations show:

Hb	183 g/l
WCC	6.6×10^9/l
RBC	6.1×10^{12}/l
Plt	317×10^9/l
MCV	88 fl
MCH	30.5 pg
MCHC	31.5 g/dl
PCV	0.48

1. Which of the following tests is likely to be normal?

- ❑ A Arterial blood gases
- ❑ B FEV_1
- ❑ C Red cell mass
- ❑ D Carboxyhaemoglobin
- ❑ E Erythropoietin

2. What is the most important step in the management?

- ❑ A Stop diuretic
- ❑ B Stop smoking
- ❑ C Venesection
- ❑ D Tight blood pressure control
- ❑ E Continue aspirin

NEPHROLOGY QUESTIONS: CASE HISTORIES

For 'best-of-five' questions candidates must select one answer only, by putting a cross in the appropriate box.

Case History 1 (9 marks)

A 66-year-old man is under investigation for backache, weight loss and intermittent low grade temperature. In the past he had a Polya gastrectomy at the age of 39 for recurrent ulcers and a right-sided renal colic ten years previously. His current medication is lisinopril and bumetanide K for moderate hypertension and warfarin which was started three years previously for transient ischaemic attacks. He is an ex-smoker and drinks approximately 25 units of alcohol per week.

Clinical examination reveals an emphysematous chest. BP 160/90 mmHg, PR 80–85/min, atrial fibrillation, 1/6 ejection systolic murmur in the aortic area and a soft right-sided carotid bruit. The liver edge is just palpable but non-tender, the spleen is not enlarged. The left testicle is tender with moderate varicocele. No lymphadenopathy is present, the CNS shows no deficit.

The following results are obtained:

Hb	179 g/l
WCC	4.7 x 10^9/l
Plt	210 x 10^9/l
PCV	0.68
ESR	70 mm/hr
INR	3.4
Na	147 mmol/l
K	3.2 mmol/l
Creatinine	178 (mol/l
Random glucose	6.8 mmol/l
Dipstix urine	Glucose -, Bilirubin - , Blood ++, Protein +
Urinary Na	48 mmol/l (60–160 mmol/l)

1. What is the likely diagnosis?

❑ A Renal artery stenosis
❑ B Renal infarction
❑ C Adrenal carcinoma
❑ D Conn's syndrome
❑ E Hypernephroma

2. What is the likely cause for the electrolyte disturbance?

- ❑ A Diuretic therapy
- ❑ B ACE-inhibitor therapy
- ❑ C Hyperaldosteronaemia
- ❑ D Hyperreninaemia
- ❑ E Reduced renal blood flow

3. What complication has apparently arisen?

- ❑ A Renal artery occlusion
- ❑ B Renal vein thrombosis
- ❑ C Renal embolization
- ❑ D Chronic renal hypoxia
- ❑ E Secondary hyperaldosteronism

While awaiting further investigations, the patient collapses with a right-sided weakness and up-going plantar. An immediate CT brain is reported as normal.

4. What cause has to be considered?

- ❑ A Hypertensive stroke
- ❑ B Significant hypotensive episode
- ❑ C Vascular occlusion due to polycythaemia
- ❑ D Embolism from right carotid plaque
- ❑ E Over-anticoagulation

Case History 2 (5 marks)

A 6-year-old boy presents with increasing shortness of breath and bilateral ankle oedema. He has previously been fit and well, except for a severe lower respiratory tract infection six months previously. On examination there is mild ankle oedema. The lungs are clear, abdomen is unremarkable. The following results are obtained:

Hb	146 g/l
WCC	5.8 x 10^9/l
Plt	318 x 10^9/l
ESR	18 mm/hr
Na	134 mmol/l
K	3.9 mmol/l
Urea	9.8 mmol/l
Creatinine	78 µmol/l
Albumin	30 g/l
Urinary protein	320 mg/24h
Dipstix urine	Blood -, Protein +++

A renal biopsy is normal on light microscopy.

1. What is the likely diagnosis?

- ❑ A IgA-nephropathy
- ❑ B Minimal change nephropathy
- ❑ C Immune complex nephritis
- ❑ D Goodpasture's syndrome
- ❑ E Crescentic glomuleronephritis

2. What therapy would you recommend?

- ❑ A Systemic steroids
- ❑ B Methotrexate
- ❑ C Cyclosporin
- ❑ D Cyclophosphamide
- ❑ E Protein supplements only

Case History 3 (8 marks)

A 48-year-old woman with SLE is on haemodialysis for end-stage renal failure. She now complains of pain in her left hand and paraesthesia over the thenar eminence which is aggravated during haemodialysis. She has her second fistula at the radial aspect of her left forearm. This had required angioplasty three months previously but has been working satisfactorily since. Her lupus is well controlled on immunosuppressants, except for a mild polyarthropathy of the small joints.

On examination, there is wasting of the thenar eminence and a 3/5 weakness of abduction and apposition of the thumb. There is also reduction of sensation to pin prick and soft touch over the tips of thumb and index finger. The following results are obtained prior to dialysis:

Hb	108 g/l
WCC	6.3 x 10^9/l
Plt	207 x 10^9/l
Na	133 mmol/l
K	5.1 mmol/l
Urea	18.5 mmol/l
Creatinine	986 µmol/l
Calcium	2.05 mmol/l
Phosphate	1.5 mmol/l
Albumin	39 g/l
Total T4	69 nmol/l (75–150 nmol/l)
TSH	2.4 mU/l

Hand X-ray shows sub-periosteal bone resorption of most phalanges, widespread arterial calcification and a well-defined lytic lesion expanding the left first metacarpal.

1. **What two complications have arisen?**
2. **Suggest two further investigations.**
3. **What treatments would you suggest?**

Case History 4 (9 marks)

A 17-year-old man is referred by the GP for investigation of haematuria. Examination of the abdomen is unremarkable. BP 165/95 mmHg, PR 72/min, regular. Despite mydriatic eye-drops, the fundi cannot be adequately assessed. In addition, a mild hearing deficit is identified and tuning-fork tests show the following results:

Weber lateralises to the right, Rinné demonstrates air conduction better than bone conduction in both ears.
Blood results in clinic are as follows:

Hb	162 g/l
WCC	5.1 x 10^9/l
Plt	265 x 10^9/l
Na	138 mmol/l
K	4.8 mmol/l
Creatinine	286 µmol/l
Dipstix urine:	Protein +, Blood ++

1. **What is the abnormality in the hearing tests?**
2. **What is the likely reason for the failed fundoscopy?**
3. **What is the diagnosis?**
4. **What is the prognosis?**

Case History 5 (5 marks)

A 23-year-old medical student on holiday in Greece became unwell with a sore throat, cervical lymphadenopathy and a low grade pyrexia. He started himself on oral amoxycillin, but three days later noticed a dark discoloration of his urine. This improved slightly with increased fluid intake, but he went to consult a local GP as there was no improvement in his symptoms after five days. He was given oral clarithromycin and after a further two days he developed abdominal pain and diarrhoea. He returned to the United Kingdom and presented to Casualty.

On examination, he has some small lymph nodes in the anterior cervical triangle. Both tonsils and Waldeyer's ring are mildly erythematous, but no pus is seen. There is tenderness in both loins but no hepato-splenomegaly. BP 175/95 mmHg, PR 88/min regular, no peripheral oedema, normal fundoscopy.

The following results were obtained:

Hb	151 g/l
WCC	8.5 x 10^9/l (58% lymphocytes)
Plt	158 x 10^9/l
ESR	24 mm/hr
Na	142 mmol/l
K	4.1 mmol/l
Urea	9.8 mmol/l
Creatinine	134 μmol/l
Urinary Na	85 mmol/l (60–160 mmol/l)
Dipstix urine	Blood +++, Protein +, Glucose +

Urine microscopy: Numerous red cells, some red cell casts

Serum C3 complement	1.25 g/l (0.55–1.20 g/l)
Serum C4 complement	0.38 g/l (0.20–0.50 g/l)

1. What is the likely diagnosis?

- ❑ A Post-streptococcal glomerulonephritis
- ❑ B Henoch-Schönlein purpura
- ❑ C Wegener's granulomatosis
- ❑ D Acute tubular necrosis
- ❑ E IgA nephropathy

2. How would you confirm the diagnosis?

- ❑ A Culture of a throat swab
- ❑ B ASO-titre
- ❑ C Renal biopsy
- ❑ D Auto-antibody screen
- ❑ E Serum IgA levels

Case History 6 (6 marks)

A 53-year-old man presents with several weeks' history of malaise and exercise dyspnoea. He returned to the UK six months' previously after having spent three years on agricultural development in Kenya. He is referred by the GP following two episodes of haemoptysis. Other than for exercise induced episodes of asthma during adolescence, the only history of note is a cholecystectomy for gallstones at the age of 42.

He is on no current medication, smokes 25 cigarettes per day but does not drink any alcohol.

On examination, he is pale with bilateral ankle oedema. Auscultation reveals bilateral basal crackles, but no heart murmur. BP 185/100 mmHg, PR 84/min, sinus rhythm. Examination of abdomen and CNS are unremarkable.

The following results are obtained:

Hb	137 g/l
WCC	5.2 x 10^9/l
Plt	109 x 10^9/l
ESR	93 mm/hr
Na	134 mmol/l
K	5.2 mmol/l
Creatinine	563 µmol/l
Total protein	53 g/l
Dipstix urine	Blood +, Protein +++, Glucose +

Renal Ultrasound: Bilaterally enlarged kidneys, without evidence of scars or hydronephrosis
Chest X-ray: Multiple ill-defined opacities in both lungs, bilateral septal lines and small pleural effusions.

1. What diagnosis is least likely?

- ❑ A Panarteritis nodosa
- ❑ B Medullary sponge kidney
- ❑ C Churg-Strauss syndrome
- ❑ D Goodpasture's syndrome
- ❑ E Membranous glomerulonephritis

A renal biopsy shows crescent formation in most glomeruli. The patient has a further episode of haemoptysis and a repeat chest X-ray shows deterioration of the previous appearances with several thick-walled cavities in both lungs. Renal angiography shows no vascular abnormality.

2. What is the likely underlying diagnosis?

- ❑ A Wegener's granulomatosis
- ❑ B Polyarteritis nodosa
- ❑ C Churg-Strauss syndrome
- ❑ D Alveoli cell carcinoma
- ❑ E Goodpasture's syndrome

3. What further investigation is likely to be diagnostic?

- ❑ A Anti-glomerular basement membrane antibodies
- ❑ B Anti-neutrophilic cytoplasmic antibodies
- ❑ C Bronchoscopy and pulmonary lavage
- ❑ D Pulmonary angiography
- ❑ E Pulmonary transfer factor (DLCO)

Case History 7 (9 marks)

A 73-year-old pensioner is referred to the Urology department with a five-month history of frequency and a two-day history of acute lower left-sided back pain. Over the last year she has lost 1.5 kg in weight and complained of increased thirst. A random blood glucose was found to be 9 mmol/l and she has been started on gliclazide 40 mg by her GP. Her only other medication was 2.5 mg bendrofluazide for mild hypertension.

Blood results on admission:

Hb	99 g/l
WCC	3.9 x 10^9/l
Plt	109 x 10^9/l
ESR	108 mm/hr
Na	144 mmol/l
K	3.2 mmol/l
Urea	11.6 mmol/l
Creatinine	168 µmol/l
Corrected calcium	3.4 mmol/l

An abdominal X-ray showed some calcification projecting over the left kidney, but an IVU performed on the same day, showed no evidence of renal obstruction.

1. **Suggest two non-invasive further investigations.**
2. **What is the likely diagnosis?**

The patient's condition deteriorates over the following two days. She becomes very dyspnoeic and requires 35% oxygen. Repeat electrolytes show the following results:

Na	145 mmol/l
K	5.8 mmol/l
Urea	28.3 mmol/l
Creatinine	612 µmol/l

3. **What complication has arisen?**
4. **What additional information is provided by this complication?**

Case History 8 (8 marks)

A 28-year-old male presents to the A&E Department with acute, right-sided flank pain.

There were no previous episodes. Brought up as a single adopted child he has always been well and never been to see his GP. He admits, however, to a one-year history of intravenous substance abuse. On examination, there are needle marks in both elbows with thrombosis of the cephalic veins. No palpable AV-fistula. BP 165/100 mmHg, PR 80/min, regular, no heart murmurs.

The liver is enlarged and an irregular mass is palpable in the left upper quadrant.

The following results are obtained:

Hb	149 g/l
WCC	3.1 x 10^9/l (84% granulocytes)
Plt	238 x 10^9/l
ESR	6 mm/hr
Na	139 mmol/l
K	4.6 mmol/l
Urea	14.1 mmol/l
Creatinine	289 μmol/l

Urine microscopy: Multiple red blood cells, several hyaline casts

IVU shows poor excretion through the left kidney, the right side shows compression of the collecting system with a splaying and elongation of the calyces.

1. What is the likely cause for the presentation?

- ❑ A Passage of renal stone
- ❑ B Acute tubular necrosis
- ❑ C Haemorrhage into cyst
- ❑ D Malignant transformation
- ❑ E Pyelonephritis

2. What is the likely diagnosis?

- ❑ A Adult polycystic disease
- ❑ B Infantile polycystic disease
- ❑ C Horseshoe kidney
- ❑ D Multicystic dysplastic kidney
- ❑ E Tuberous sclerosis

Pulse oximetry reveals an oxygen saturation of 95% on room air and chest X-ray shows bilateral diffuse mid-zone shadowing. On moderate exercise, the patient de-saturates to 85%.

3. What diagnosis has to be considered?

- ❑ A Interstitial pulmonary oedema
- ❑ B Sarcoidosis
- ❑ C Pulmonary haemorrhage
- ❑ D *Pneumocystis carinii* pneumonia
- ❑ E Eosinophilic pneumonia

With treatment, the patient makes a good recovery but is lost to follow-up. Eight months later he is brought back to the A&E Department after having been found collapsed on a park bench. On examination, he has a Glasgow Coma Scale of 5 with flexion to pain stimulus. An un-enhanced CT of the brain is reported as normal.

A lumbar puncture reveals the following results:

Opening pressure	14 cm H_2O
Xanthochromia	++
Protein	0.28 g/l (0.2–0.4 g/l)
Glucose	59% of blood glucose
Microscopy	4 red cells/μl (< 5 per μl)

4. What is the likely explanation for these results?

- ❑ A Traumatic tap
- ❑ B Haemorrhagic stroke
- ❑ C Herpes encephalitis
- ❑ D Cerebral toxoplasmosis
- ❑ E Subarachnoid haemorrhage

NEPHROLOGY QUESTIONS: DATA INTERPRETATIONS

For 'best-of-five' questions candidates must select one answer only, by putting a cross in the appropriate box.

Data Interpretation 1 (3 marks)

A diet-controlled Type II diabetic is admitted with blunt abdominal trauma following a road traffic accident. He is stabilised with conservative management, but a day later shows the following blood results:

Na	142 mmol/l
K	5.5 mmol/l
Chloride	98 mmol/l
Bicarbonate	19.5 mmol/l
Urea	16 mmol/l
Creatinine	196 µmol/l
Glucose	13 mmol/l
Dipstix urine	Blood ++, Protein -, Ketones + Glucose ++

1. What is the likely cause for these results?

❑ A Renal contusion
❑ B Ketoacidosis
❑ C Lactic acidosis Type A
❑ D Lactic acidosis Type B
❑ E Rhabdomyolysis

Data Interpretation 2 (4 marks)

Following an episode of gastroenteritis, a 7-year-old child is admitted extremely unwell with the following blood results:

Hb	132 g/l
MCV	99 fl
WCC	7.2 x 10^9/l
Plt	87 x 10^9/l
Blood film: 9% reticulocytes, multiple schistocytes and fragmentocytes	
Na	138 mmol/l
K	5.2 mmol/l
Creatinine	216 μmol/l

1. What is the likely diagnosis?

- ❑ A Reiter's syndrome
- ❑ B Henoch-Schönlein purpura
- ❑ C Idiopathic thrombocytopaenic purpura
- ❑ D Acute sickle-cell crisis
- ❑ E Haemolytic uraemic syndrome

2. What is the likely precipitating cause?

- ❑ A Dehydration
- ❑ B Hypoxia
- ❑ C *E. coli* infection
- ❑ D Parvovirus B19 infection
- ❑ E Methanol ingestion

Data Interpretation 3 (2 marks)

These are the arterial blood gases of a 69-year-old woman with chronic obstructive airways disease (COAD) (room air).

pH	7.21
pO_2	6.8 kPa
pCO_2	7.9 kPa
HCO_3^-	18 mmol/l
O_2-saturation	87%

1. What is the best way to describe these results?

- ❑ A Respiratory acidosis
- ❑ B Combined respiratory and metabolic acidosis
- ❑ C Combined respiratory acidosis and metabolic alkalosis
- ❑ D Venous sample
- ❑ E Laboratory error

Data Interpretation 4 (4 marks)

A 29-year-old woman is under investigation for renal colic. These are her blood results:

Na	139 mmol/l
K	2.8 mmol/l
Urea	6.3 mmol/l
Creatinine	131 µmol/l
Bicarbonate	13 mmol/l
Calcium	2.0 mmol/l
Phosphate	0.8 mmol/l
Albumin	29 mmol/l
Total protein	59 g/l
AST	95 U/l

1. **What is the likely diagnosis?**
2. **Suggest a precipitating cause.**

Data Interpretation 5 (4 marks)

A 46-year-old woman had a pan-proctocolectomy for ulcerative colitis at the age of 38. She now presents with symptoms of an acute left renal colic. A plain abdominal radiograph shows no evidence of stones. Ultrasound of the kidneys shows no evidence of hydronephrosis. The following blood results are obtained:

Na	141 mmol/l
K	3.6 mmol/l
Urea	7.8 mmol/l
Bicarbonate	18 mmol/l
Albumin	31 g/l
Calcium	2.2 mmol/l
Phosphate	0.85 mmol/l

1. What is the most likely diagnosis?

- ❑ A Renal papillary necrosis
- ❑ B Urate stones
- ❑ C Oxalate stones
- ❑ D Retroperitoneal fibrosis
- ❑ E Ureteric stricture

2. What treatment would you suggest?

- ❑ A Ureteric stent
- ❑ B Extracorporeal lithotripsy
- ❑ C Balloon dilatation
- ❑ D Bicarbonate supplements
- ❑ E Urine acidification

Data Interpretation 6 (3 marks)

A 2-year-old child is being investigated for irritability associated with a low grade pyrexia. On examination, the patient has a right upper quadrant mass. The following blood results are obtained:

Hb	107 g/l
WCC	5.9×10^9/l
Plt	241×10^9/l
ESR	12 mm/hr
Na	143 mmol/l
K	3.8 mmol/l
Creatinine	65 µmol/l
Dipstix urine	Blood +, Protein -, Glucose -
Urine microscopy	
Red cells	15/µl (<5/µl)
White cells	8/µl (<10/µl)
Several granular casts	

1. What is the likely diagnosis?

- ❑ A Wilms' tumour
- ❑ B Horseshoe kidney
- ❑ C Crossed fused ectopia
- ❑ D Vesico-ureteric reflux
- ❑ E Infantile polycystic disease

Data Interpretation 7 (4 marks)

A 53-year-old woman with long-standing active rheumatoid arthritis presents with shortness of breath and tiredness. Blood samples show the following results:

Hb	78 g/l
WCC	1.9 x 10^9/l
Plt	57 x 10^9/l
ESR	57 mm/hr
Na	141 mmol/l
K	3.2 mmol/l
Albumin	25 g/l
Urinary protein	2.8 g/24hr

Renal biopsy shows diffuse thickening of the glomerular basement membrane.

1. What is the likely mechanism for the abnormality in the blood count?

❑ A Aplastic anaemia
❑ B Haemolytic anaemia
❑ C Anaemia of chronic disease
❑ D Folate deficiency
❑ E Sideroblastic anaemia

2. What is the cause for the renal abnormality?

❑ A Small vessel vasculitis
❑ B Immune complex deposition
❑ C Analgesic nephropathy
❑ D Drug-induced glomerulonephritis
❑ E Papillary necrosis

Data Interpretation 8 (4 marks)

A 48-year-old unemployed electrician is admitted to Casualty after being found unconscious at a building site. His vital signs are stable, the following results are obtained:

Na	132 mmol/l
K	6.9 mmol/l
Urea	16.2 mmol/l
Creatinine	821 μmol/l
ALT	53 U/l
AST	348 U/l
Uristix	Blood +++, Protein +, Ketones -

1. **What do these results suggest?**
2. **What is the likely precipitating cause?**

Data Interpretation 9 (4 marks)

A medical referral is made from the psychiatric unit about a 23-year-old man with deteriorating renal function and acute arthritis in the right foot. The only family history of note is schizophrenia of the maternal grandfather who committed suicide at the age of 29. The following results are obtained:

Na	138 mmol/l
K	4.9 mmol/l
Urea	16.3 mmol/l
Creatinine	437 µmol/l
Bicarbonate	20 mmol/l

An X-ray of his foot shows areas of soft tissue calcification and punched out juxta-articular erosions around the interphalangeal joints.

1. What is the likely diagnosis?

❑ A Variegate porphyria
❑ B Gout nephropathy
❑ C Lithium toxicity
❑ D Lesch-Nyhan syndrome
❑ E Exacerbation of psoriatic arthropathy

2. What is the underlying mechanism?

❑ A Increased cell turnover
❑ B X-linked recessive enzyme defect
❑ C Autosomal recessive liver defect
❑ D Chronic haemolytic anaemia
❑ E Familial tubular defect

Data Interpretation 10 (6 marks)

A 49-year-old woman with systemic lupus erythyematodes is under follow-up for membranous glomerulonephritis. Her previously impaired, but stable renal function has deteriorated rapidly over the space of a week. Investigations reveal:

Na	138 mmol/l
K	5.8 mmol/l
Urea	38 mmol/l
Creatinine	1,000 µmol/l
Albumin	19 g/l
Urinary protein	18 g/24h
Dipstix urine	Blood ++, Protein +++

1. **What is the most likely diagnosis?**
2. **What treatment would you suggest?**
3. **What is the prognosis regarding the renal function?**

Data Interpretation 11 (5 marks)

A 32-year-old man is referred to clinic after an insurance medical revealed hypertension. The following results are obtained:

Na	145 mmol/l
K	Haemolysed
Bicarbonate	32 mmol/l
Creatinine	131 μmol/l
Urinary Na	48 mmol/l (< 40 mmol/l)

The following results are obtained after 25 mg oral captopril.

Time [min]	**0**	**120**
Aldosterone [80–400 pmol/l]	489	280
Renin [3–19 ng/l]	21	48

1. What is the diagnosis?

- ❑ A Essential hypertensive
- ❑ B Conn's syndrome
- ❑ C Renal artery stenosis
- ❑ D Adreno-cortical hyperplasia
- ❑ E Renin-secreting tumour

2. What treatment would you suggest?

- ❑ A ACE-inhibitors
- ❑ B Loop diuretics
- ❑ C Angiotensin receptor blockers
- ❑ D Renal artery angioplasty
- ❑ E Adrenalectomy

Data Interpretation 12 (5 marks)

A 23-year-old Turkish women presents with malaise, weight loss and polyuria. The following results are obtained:

Na	127 mmol/l
K	4.1 mmol/l
Urea	8.1 mmol/l
Creatinine	117 μmol/l
Urine microscopy	
Red cells	8/μl (< 5/μl)
White cells	95/μl (< 10/μl)
Multiple hyaline casts	
Urinary Na excretion	410 mmol/24 hr (40–220 mmol/24 hr)
MSU x 3	No growth

1. What is the cause for the electrolyte imbalance?

- ❑ A Pyelonephritis
- ❑ B Acute tubular necrosis
- ❑ C Salt-wasting nephropathy
- ❑ D Nephrogenic diabetes insipidus
- ❑ E Inappropriate ADH secretion

2. What is the likely underlying cause?

- ❑ A Gonorrhoea
- ❑ B Vesico-ureteric reflux
- ❑ C Chlamydia infection
- ❑ D Fanconi's syndrome
- ❑ E Renal tuberculosis

Data Interpretation 13 (4 marks)

A 32-year-old woman is under investigation for dysuria and secondary infertility. She also complains of polyarthralgia and sharp pains in the right upper quadrant. The following results are obtained:

Hb	129 g/l
WCC	8.9 x 10^9/l
Plt	328 x 10^9/l
ESR	56 mm/hr
Na	138 mmol/l
K	4.1 mmol/l
Creatinine	92 µmol/l
Albumin	42 g/l
Dipstix urine	Blood +, White cells ++
Midstream urine culture	Negative

1. What is your next investigation?

- ❑ A Pelvic ultrasound
- ❑ B Hystero-salpingography
- ❑ C Blood culture
- ❑ D Cervical swab
- ❑ E Liver function tests

2. What is the likely diagnosis?

- ❑ A Gonorrhoea
- ❑ B Chlamydia infection
- ❑ C Endometriosis
- ❑ D Reiter's syndrome
- ❑ E Behçet syndrome

Data Interpretation 14 (4 marks)

A retired chemical worker presents with intermittent right loin pain. Clinical examination is unremarkable, he is on enalapril 10 mg and aspirin 150 mg. Blood results show:

Na	139 mmol/l
K	4.0 mmol/l
Urea	9.3 mmol/l
Creatinine	165 μmol/l
Calcium	2.6 mmol/l
Albumin	41 g/l
Bilirubin	18 μmol/l
Alkaline phosphatase	320 U/l
Urine microscopy	
Red cells	15/μl (< 5/μl)
White cells	8/μl (< 10/μl)
No casts	

1. What two investigations would you perform next?

- ❑ A Uric acid levels and cystoscopy
- ❑ B Captopril test and chest X-ray
- ❑ C DMSA renogram and serum bicarbonate
- ❑ D Urine electrolytes and renal angiography
- ❑ E Urine cytology and radio-isotope bone scan

2. What is the likely underlying cause?

- ❑ A Transitional cell carcinoma
- ❑ B Hemangioblastoma
- ❑ C Renal artery stenosis
- ❑ D Retroperitoneal fibrosis
- ❑ E Prostatic carcinoma

Data Interpretation 15 (5 marks)

A 68-year-old woman presents to the GP with low back pain (relieved by rest) and bilateral knee pain. She is given painkillers, but presents five weeks later to the Casualty Department with orthopnoea, bilateral leg oedema and clinical evidence of ascites. Immediate results show:

Na	143 mmol/l
K	5.6 mmol/l
Creatinine	199 μmol/l
Dipstix urine	Glucose ++, Protein +++, Blood +, Ketones -

1. What is the most likely diagnosis?

- ❑ A Renal vein thrombosis
- ❑ B Allergic interstitial nephritis
- ❑ C Renal papillary necrosis
- ❑ D Analgesic nephropathy
- ❑ E Acute tubular necrosis

2. What treatment would you suggest?

- ❑ A Oral steroids
- ❑ B Cyclosporin
- ❑ C Forced diuresis
- ❑ D Anticoagulation
- ❑ E Withdrawal of all medication

Data Interpretation 16 (4 marks)

A 43-year-old salesman presents after two years in the Far East with a macular erythematous rash, lymphadenopathy and painless buccal ulcers. On examination, he has a low grade pyrexia with evidence of meningism. He is admitted as an emergency and given intravenous penicillin.

1. What investigation is likely to be diagnostic?

- ❑ A Blood culture
- ❑ B Lumbar puncture
- ❑ C Oral swab and dark field microscopy
- ❑ D *Treponema pallidum* haemagglutination test
- ❑ E Viral serology

The following day, the patient becomes extremely unwell with fever, polymyalgia and hypotension.

2. What complication has occurred?

- ❑ A Waterhouse-Friderichsen syndrome
- ❑ B Jarisch-Herxheimer reaction
- ❑ C Anaphylactic reaction to penicillin
- ❑ D Stevens-Johnson syndrome
- ❑ E Septicaemia

NEUROLOGY QUESTIONS: CASE HISTORIES

For 'best-of-five' questions candidates must select one answer only, by putting a cross in the appropriate box.

Case History 1 (7 marks)

A 73-year-old man is admitted to the A&E Department with weakness of his left arm and leg. He has a history of atrial fibrillation and was anticoagulated two years previously after several TIA's affecting his right arm. Three weeks prior to admission, his General Practitioner was called to see him because he had become unrousable. He had recovered by the time the GP arrived and had no residual neurological signs. Since then, however, he has been experiencing difficulties in concentrating and has become unsteady on his feet. His current medication is digoxin 125 μg, enalapril 10 mg and warfarin.

On examination he is alert but disorientated to time and place. BP 185/100 mmHg, PR 88/min, irregular. There is a soft, left-sided carotid bruit and a flow murmur in the aortic area. He has a 4/5 pyramidal weakness affecting the left arm and leg with extensor response in both plantars. There is no papilloedema, examination of chest and abdomen are unremarkable.

While recording an ECG, a nurse observes the patient becoming drowsy and unresponsive to speech, however when re-examined by the House Officer 10 minutes later he is fully alert again with no change in clinical signs. During that episode he has been incontinent of urine.

Investigations reveal:

Hb	142 g/l
WCC	5.3 x 10^9/l
Plt	177 x 10^9/l
ESR	16 mm/hr
Na	130 mmol/l
K	3.5 mmol/l
Urea	3.0 mmol/l
Creatinine	127 μmol/l

ECG: controlled atrial fibrillation, 1 mm ST depression in lateral chest leads.

1. Which of the following investigations is unlikely to be helpful?

- ❑ A Prothrombin time
- ❑ B Blood glucose
- ❑ C Carotid Doppler
- ❑ D Serum and urine osmolality
- ❑ E Brain CT

2. What is the likely diagnosis?

- ❑ A Vertebro-basilar insufficiency
- ❑ B Right middle cerebral artery emboli
- ❑ C Cerebral metastases
- ❑ D Colloid cyst of third ventricle
- ❑ E Chronic subdural haematoma

3. Which of the following management options would be the most appropriate?

- ❑ A Neurosurgical referral
- ❑ B iv dexamethasone
- ❑ C Radiotherapy
- ❑ D Add oral aspirin
- ❑ E Increase warfarin

Case History 2 (8 marks)

A 23-year-old architecture student from Morocco is referred by his GP. Over the last six weeks he has become unsteady on his feet and now finds it impossible to keep his balance in the dark. The only past medical history of note is enucleation of his right eye at the age of 12 for a 'growth'.

On examination he is ataxic with a positive Romberg's test. Nystagmus is present in both eyes which is not affected by posture and there is no definite associated vertigo. There is mild dysdiadochokinesis in the right hand. Examination of the cranial nerves and the remainder of the peripheral nervous system reveals no further abnormalities. The blood pressure is elevated at 190/110 mmHg with an ejection murmur over the aortic area.

The liver is not enlarged but a mass can be balloted in the left upper quadrant.

The following results are obtained:

Hb	186 g/l
WCC	6.1 x 10^9/l
Plt	216 x 10^9/l
ESR	2 mm/hr
MCV	73 fl
Hkt	61%
Na	136 mmol/l
K	4.1 mmol/l
Urea	6.2 mmol/l
Creatinine	81 μmol/l
Albumin	42 g/l
Dipstix urine	Blood ++, Protein -, Bilirubin -

Ultrasound abdomen: 8 cm inhomogeneous mass left kidney, 2 cm nodule lower pole right kidney, several liver cysts

1. What is your next investigation?

- ❑ A Chest X-ray
- ❑ B Intravenous urogram
- ❑ C Urinary catecholamine levels
- ❑ D Erythropoietin levels
- ❑ E CT abdomen

A CT scan of the brain shows two cystic nodules within the cerebellum. No supra-tentorial lesions are identified.

2. What is the underlying diagnosis?

- ❑ A Malignant melanoma of uvea
- ❑ B Rhabdomyosarcoma of orbit
- ❑ C von Hippel-Lindau syndrome
- ❑ D Tuberose sclerosis
- ❑ E Neurofibromatosis Type II

3. What are the renal lesions?

- ❑ A Metastases
- ❑ B Haematomata
- ❑ C Bilateral phaeochromocytomata
- ❑ D Bilateral renal cell carcinomata
- ❑ E Neurofibromata

The patient enquires whether there is a particular risk of his two-month-old son developing the same problem.

4. How do you estimate the risk?

- ❑ A No increased risk
- ❑ B 25%
- ❑ C 40–50%
- ❑ D 66%
- ❑ E 92–100%

Case History 3 (7 marks)

A 23-year-old man presents to the A&E Department with a one week history of increasing malaise and tiredness. In addition, he has experienced increasing difficulties in walking and in the last two days has had problems feeding himself, with liquid dribbling from the corners of his mouth.

On examination he has a mild ptosis of his left eye and is unable to whistle. Reduced tone is present in the legs and limb weakness is noted. Power is reduced to 3/5 for ankle extension and to 4/5 for knee and wrist extension. The ankle jerks are absent, knee and biceps jerks are present with reinforcement. There is reduced sensation to pinprick and soft touch to the level of both knees and the fingertips of the right hand. Fundoscopy reveals mild swelling of the right disc. Blood pressure 125/70 mmHg, pulse 96/min, regular. Respiratory rate 24/min, normal breath sounds on auscultation. Examination of the abdomen is unremarkable.

The following results are obtained:

Hb	146 g/l
WCC	6.2×10^9/l
Plt	193×10^9/l
ESR	13 mm/hr
Biochemical profile	Normal
Glucose	5.8 mmol/l

The following CSF results are obtained at lumbar puncture:

Opening pressure	24 cm H_2O
Protein	2.3 g/l
Glucose	4.9 mmol/l
Microscopy	6 lymphocytes/mm^3, no polymorphs
Peroneal nerve conduction velocity	21 m/s (> 45 m/s)

1. What is the likely diagnosis?

- ❑ A Tetanus
- ❑ B Guillain-Barré syndrome
- ❑ C Botulism
- ❑ D Multiple sclerosis
- ❑ E Herpes simplex encephalitis

2. Which further investigation is indicated?

- ❑ A Chest X-ray
- ❑ B CT brain
- ❑ C Pulmonary function tests
- ❑ D Clostridium serology
- ❑ E Visual evoked potentials

3. What treatment has to be considered?

- ❑ A im anti-toxin
- ❑ B Ventilation
- ❑ C iv interferon
- ❑ D Pyridostigmine
- ❑ E iv penicillin

Case History 4 (7 marks)

A 4-year-old boy is referred from the GP with shortness of breath on exercise and unwillingness to play with his friends. This has come on over the previous six months after initially normal developmental milestones. When called into the examination room, he needs support from his mother to get up from the floor.

Examination shows a mentally normally developed child. He is short of breath at rest, examination of chest and cardiovascular system are otherwise unremarkable. He has very well developed calves, but a symmetrical moderate weakness of the pelvic and shoulder girdle are present.

Investigations show:

Hb	138 g/l
WCC	5.2 x 10^9/l
Plt	327 x 10^9/l
ESR	8 mm/hr
Na	134 mmol/l
K	4.9 mmol/l
Urea	4.1 mmol/l
Albumin	38 g/l
Chest X-ray	Mild cardiomegaly

Electromyography shows polyphasic action potentials of short duration and low amplitude.

1. **What is the likely diagnosis?**
2. **Suggest a further investigation.**
3. **What is the prognosis?**

Case History 5 (7 marks)

The 49-year-old wife of a publican presents to the Outpatient Department with a several week history of difficulties walking. She also complains of annoying paraesthesia of the toes and fingertips which has been worse at night. She also gives a six month history of tiredness and finding it difficult to cope with her daily tasks. At the age of 28 she had been successfully treated for lymphoma. Her current medication consists of bezafibrate for a raised cholesterol and folate prescribed by her GP. She smokes 20 cigarettes per day and suffers from a chronic, productive cough. Alcohol intake is 15–20 units per week.

On examination she is pale with a blood pressure of 155/90 mmHg. No murmurs. There are bi-basal crackles on auscultation, improved after coughing. In the abdomen a smooth liver edge is palpable without splenomegaly or lymphadenopathy.

In the legs there is a 4/5 weakness at the knees and ankles. Both knee-jerks are brisk and several beats of clonus can be elicited at the patellae, however, there is reduced tone at the ankles and the ankle-jerks are absent. Both plantar responses are extensor. Vibration sense is absent at the ankle and reduced at the knee, there is reduced sensation to pinprick below the ankle. Mild paraesthesia is present in the fingertips, no significant abnormality is found otherwise in the upper limbs. No cerebellar signs can be elicited.

The following results are obtained:

Hb	102 g/l
WCC	3.8 x 10^9/l
Plt	106 x 10^9/l
ESR	23 mm/hr
Na	139 mmol/l
K	4.1 mmol/l
Creatinine	138 µmol/l
Albumin	44 g/l
AST	26 U/l

Nerve conduction studies:

Sural sensory action potential	4 µV (> 50 µV)
Peroneal nerve conduction velocity	49 m/s (> 45 m/s)

1. Which of the following investigations is likely to be of diagnostic value?

- ❑ A Chest X-ray
- ❑ B Blood film
- ❑ C Red cell transketolase
- ❑ D MR scan of brain
- ❑ E MR scan of spine

2. What is the diagnosis?

- ❑ A Subacute combined degeneration of the cord
- ❑ B Tabes dorsalis
- ❑ C Hereditary sensory-motor neuropathy
- ❑ D Eaton-Lambert syndrome
- ❑ E Toxic neuropathy

3. Which of the following may worsen the condition?

- ❑ A Alcohol withdrawal
- ❑ B Bed rest
- ❑ C Folate replacement
- ❑ D Antibiotic therapy
- ❑ E Physiotherapy

Case History 6 (8 marks)

A 53-year-old female office clerk is referred by the GP for investigation of diplopia and a proximal muscle weakness. Her symptoms are worst in the morning and tend to improve through the day. In addition she complains of a three month history of malaise and a weight gain of 1.5 kg.

On examination there is wasting of both thighs and upper arms with reduction of power at the hip flexors of 3/5 and at the deltoid of 4/5. She is unable to stand up from a squatting position, biceps and knee-jerks are reduced and the ankle-jerks are only present with reinforcement. Plantars are down-going. No motor deficit can be identified in the cranial nerves, but a mild dysarthria is present. There is a general reduction in tone. Co-ordination and sensation are normal.

The chest is clear, no heart murmurs, BP 180/105 mmHg, pulse 84/min, regular. Examination of the abdomen is difficult due to adiposity, but no organomegaly can be identified.

The following results are obtained:

Hb	109 g/l
WCC	5.7 x 10^9/l
Plt	247 x 10^9/l
MCV	73 fl
ESR	31 mm/hr
Na	146 mmol/l
K	3.1 mmol/l
Urea	8.1 mmol/l
Creatinine	139 µmol/l
Random glucose	10.8 mmol/l

1. What is the likely cause for the neurological deficit?

- ❑ A Motor neurone disease
- ❑ B Myasthenia gravis
- ❑ C Polymyositis
- ❑ D Endocrine myopathy
- ❑ E Paraneoplastic syndrome

2. How would you confirm this?

- ❑ A Muscle biopsy
- ❑ B Electromyography
- ❑ C Sural nerve biopsy
- ❑ D Response to exercise
- ❑ E Tensilon® test

3. What is the likely underlying cause for the abnormal biochemistry results?

- ❑ A Nelson's syndrome
- ❑ B Islet cell tumour
- ❑ C Ectopic ACTH secretion
- ❑ D Multiple endocrine neoplasia Type I
- ❑ E Thrombosis of IVC

4. What is the most important next investigation?

- ❑ A Chest X-ray
- ❑ B Muscle biopsy
- ❑ C Early morning cortisol
- ❑ D Auto-antibody screen
- ❑ E CT abdomen

Case History 7 (9 marks)

A 49-year-old bachelor is admitted to the Casualty Department with a one day history of worsening diplopia, blurred vision and shortness of breath. This had been preceded by diarrhoea and vomiting. A keen gardener, he had previously been fit and well, keeping himself healthy with work on his allotment and buying organic produce from the local farm. In the past he had rheumatic fever at the age of eight and suffered a basal skull fracture three years previously falling out of a cherry tree. He is on no regular medication.

On examination the patient is extremely agitated. There is a mild convergent strabismus in both eyes with poor abduction, the pupils are of normal size but show very sluggish response to light. He has difficulty swallowing his saliva and there is a moderate, global reduction in tone and power (3/5) and the reflexes are markedly depressed.

The chest is clear. A rumbling mid-systolic murmur is heard over the cardiac apex, BP 175/70 mmHg, pulse 92/min, regular.

Liver and spleen are not enlarged, but a smooth, firm mass is palpated in the lower abdomen arising from the pelvis. The patient is apyrexial but tachypnoeic at 28/min.

The following results are obtained:

Hb	142 g/l
WCC	6.1 x 10^9/l
Plt	329 x 10^9/l
Na	142 mmol/l
K	4.1 mmol/l
Creatinine	119 µmol/l
Albumin	39 g/l
Random glucose	5.9 mmol/l
C-reactive protein	7.9 mg/l (< 10mg/l)

ECG: Sinus rhythm, complete left-bundle-branch block, axis -45°, 1 mm ST depression in V5 and V6.

1. What is the likely diagnosis?

- ❑ A Botulism
- ❑ B Tetanus
- ❑ C Organophosphate poisoning
- ❑ D Rabies
- ❑ E Cerebral abscess

2. Which of the following investigations is the most important?

- ❑ A CT-brain
- ❑ B Arterial blood gases
- ❑ C Blood cultures
- ❑ D Toxicology screen
- ❑ E Viral serology

3. Which of the following should be administered?

- ❑ A iv benzyl-penicillin
- ❑ B iv gentamycin
- ❑ C Depolarising muscle relaxant
- ❑ D Atropine
- ❑ E Anti-toxin

4. What further measures are indicated?

- ❑ A Inspect patient for bite wounds and inform local council
- ❑ B Stool cultures and referral of involved staff to Occupational Health
- ❑ C Neurosurgical referral and screening of immediate relatives
- ❑ D Admit to intensive care and inform Public Health
- ❑ E Saliva samples and barrier nursing of patient

Case History 8 (9 marks)

A 29-year-old woman is referred to the Neurology Department with a recent onset of difficulties walking and dull backache. She seems to relate this to an accident three weeks previously where she was knocked off her bike. She had suffered blunt trauma to her thoracic spine, but X-rays performed in the A&E Department did not demonstrate a fracture. She was otherwise well and took no regular medication.

Examination of the upper limbs is normal. In the left leg the reflexes are brisk and several beats of clonus can be elicited at the ankle. Pin prick sensation is normal but sensation to deep pain is reduced. Power deficit of 4/5 is present in the extension of the knee.

The only deficit noticeable in the right leg is a mild reduction in pin prick over the anterior tibia and thigh to the groin with some hyperaesthesia along the right costal margins.

1. What do these findings suggest?

❑ A Left-sided disc prolapse
❑ B Right-sided thoracic tumour
❑ C Right-sided disc prolapse
❑ D Thoracic syrinx
❑ E Left-sided thoracic tumour

It is also noted that the patient has a mild convergent squint in the left eye and on formal examination there is a deficit in abduction and elevation of gaze on the left, as well as a mild mydriasis. There is no proptosis and the eyes are not injected.

2. Which of the following processes is most likely to cause this deficit?

❑ A Mononeuritis multiplex
❑ B Extradural haemorrhage
❑ C Superior orbital fissure meningioma
❑ D Cerebello pontine angle tumour
❑ E Cavernous sinus thrombosis

On further testing of the cranial nerves, a hearing deficit is detected. Testing with a tuning fork reveals the following results:

Weber: lateralising to the left
Rinné: positive in both ears (air conduction better than bone conduction)

3. What is indicated by these results?

- ❑ A Right sensory-neural deficit
- ❑ B Left sensory-neural deficit
- ❑ C Left conduction deficit
- ❑ D Right conduction deficit
- ❑ E Otosclerosis

4. Which of the following diagnoses has to be considered?

- ❑ A Multiple sclerosis
- ❑ B Basal skull fracture
- ❑ C Benign intracranial hypertension
- ❑ D Neurofibromatosis Type II
- ❑ E von Hippel-Lindau syndrome

NEUROLOGY QUESTIONS: DATA INTERPRETATIONS

For 'best-of-five' questions candidates must select one answer only, by putting a cross in the appropriate box.

Data Interpretation 1 (4 marks)

A Polish tourist presents to the A&E Department with headache, ataxia and diplopia on left lateral gaze. The following results are obtained:

Hb	135 g/l
WCC	10 x 10^9/l (59% granulocytes)
Plt	277 x 10^9/l
Glucose	5.6 mmol/l

A lumbar puncture is performed with the following results:

Opening pressure	29 cm H_2O
Protein	2.1 g/l
Glucose	0.7 mmol/l
Microscopy	125 cells/mm^3 (90% lymphocytes)

1. What is the likely diagnosis?

❑ A Viral meningitis
❑ B Herpes encephalitis
❑ C Cerebral toxoplasmosis
❑ D Tuberculous meningitis
❑ E Cerebral cysticercosis

2. What complication has arisen?

❑ A Sinus cavernosus thrombosis
❑ B Subdural empyema
❑ C Brain stem abscess
❑ D Communicating hydrocephalus
❑ E Obstructive hydrocephalus

Data Interpretation 2 (4 marks)

Following a night on the town, a 15-year old boy is admitted with speech impairment and difficulty swallowing. There is a generalised reduction in tone, power and reflexes. Sensation is normal. The following results are obtained:

Na	142 mmol/l
K	2.7 mmol/l
Urea	6.1 mmol/l
Creatinine	85 µmol/l
Glucose	6.2 mmol/l
ECG	Normal
Chest X-ray	Normal
Dipstix urine	Protein +, Glucose -, Blood -

1. Which of the following investigations would you recommend?

❑ A Electromyography
❑ B Nerve conduction studies
❑ C CT brain
❑ D Lumbar puncture
❑ E Drug screen

2. What is the likely diagnosis?

❑ A Ecstasy overdose
❑ B Periodic paralysis
❑ C McArdle's syndrome
❑ D Cocaine overdose
❑ E Myasthenia gravis

Data Interpretation 3 (5 marks)

A 36-year old woman presents with a right-sided facial weakness with inability to close the right eye. There is mild swelling of the right cheek. A lumbar puncture reveals:

Opening pressure	12 cm H_2O
Protein	0.8 g/l
Glucose	3.8 mmol/l
	(blood glucose 4.3 mmol/l)
Microscopy (/mm^3)	85 lymphocytes, 2 erythrocytes

1. Which of the following is the most likely diagnosis?

- ❑ A Bell's palsy
- ❑ B Cerebral sarcoid
- ❑ C Ramsay-Hunt syndrome
- ❑ D Right acoustic neuroma
- ❑ E Pleomorphic adenoma of parotid

2. Which of the following investigations would you perform?

- ❑ A Chest X-ray
- ❑ B CT scan of brain
- ❑ C Viral serology
- ❑ D Visual evoked potentials
- ❑ E Ultrasound scan of parotid

Data Interpretation 4 (6 marks)

A woman in her thirties is admitted from a night club having collapsed. A lobulated mass is palpated under the left costal margin.

An un-enhanced CT brain is normal. The following results are obtained:

Na	136 mmol/l
K	5.6 mmol/l
Urea	15 mmol/l
Creatinine	231 μmol/l

The following day a lumbar puncture is performed, during which the patient has a fit.

CSF shows Blood staining +, Xanthochromia ++

Pressure	17 cm H_2O
Protein	0.5 g/l
Glucose	4.2 mmol/l
Microscopy (/mm^3)	360 erythrocytes, 7 lymphocytes

1. What do the CSF results imply?

- ❑ A Traumatic tap
- ❑ B Haemorrhagic stroke
- ❑ C Subarachnoid haemorrhage
- ❑ D Ruptured arterio-venous malformation
- ❑ E Cerebral metastases

2. What is the underlying condition?

- ❑ A von Hippel-Lindau syndrome
- ❑ B Renal cell carcinoma
- ❑ C Sturge-Weber syndrome
- ❑ D Adult polycystic kidney disease
- ❑ E Hereditary haemorrhagic telangiectasia

3. What is the most sensible investigation?

- ❑ A CT brain after iv contrast
- ❑ B Ultrasound abdomen
- ❑ C Intravenous urogram
- ❑ D MAG-3 renogram
- ❑ E MR scan of brain

Data Interpretation 5 (5 marks)

A 32-year-old man is admitted to the A&E Department insisting that he has eaten 'forbidden food' and that 'the evil spirits are trying to explode his bowel'. He has peritonism with increased bowel sounds and he seems oblivious to pin prick below mid-calf. Despite fierce resistance, he is fairly easily restrained and blood samples show the following results:

Hb	151 g/l
WCC	12.2 x 10^9/l (88% neutrophils)
Plt	253 x 10^9/l
Na	127 mmol/l
K	4.8 mmol/l
Creatinine	99 µmol/l
CRP	3 mg/l

1. **What is the likely diagnosis?**

❑ A Familial Mediterranean fever
❑ B Amphetamine overdose
❑ C Hypoglycaemia
❑ D General paralysis of the insane
❑ E Acute intermittent porphyria

2. **What drug would you use for sedation?**

❑ A Midazolam
❑ B Nalbuphine
❑ C Phenobarbitone
❑ D Chlorpromazine
❑ E Diazemuls

Data Interpretation 6 (6 marks)

A 17-year-old African student presents with confusion and pyrexia. There are no focal signs, the following results are obtained:

Hb	136 g/l
WCC	17×10^9/l (12% lymphocytes)
Plt	561×10^9/l
ESR	79 mm/hr
Glucose	6.2 mmol/l

A lumbar puncture reveals:

Opening pressure	29 cm H_2O, turbid fluid
Protein	1.3 g/l
Glucose	2.6 mmol/l
Microscopy	230 cells/mm^3 (86% polymorphonuclear cells)
Gram stain	Gram positive diplococci

1. **What is the likely diagnosis?**
2. **What is the treatment?**
3. **Give two further important steps in the management.**

Data Interpretation 7 (6 marks)

An unemployed 42-year-old labourer presents with difficulties walking and palpitations. He has wasting of the facial muscles, bilateral ptosis and a distal muscle weakness. The sexual characteristics are under-developed. Visual acuity is 3/6 with glasses.

The following results are obtained:

Full blood count — Normal
Urea and electrolytes — Normal

The following blood glucose levels are obtained after oral administration of 75g disaccharides:

0 minutes	7 mmol/l
60 minutes	9.5 mmol/l
120 minutes	10.1 mmol/l

Testosterone — 6 nmol/l (12–30 nmol/l)
LH — 27 µmol/l (2–10 µmol/l)

ECG
PR 0.38 seconds
QRS 0.13 seconds
QT 0.4 seconds

1. What does the oral glucose tolerance test indicate?

- ❏ A Normal results
- ❏ B Chronic liver disease
- ❏ C Glucagonoma
- ❏ D Impaired glucose tolerance
- ❏ E Vomiting during test

2. What do the sex hormone levels suggest?

- ❑ A Hypogonadotrophic hypogonadism
- ❑ B Hypergonadotropic hypogonadism
- ❑ C Thalamic dysfunction
- ❑ D Androgen resistance
- ❑ E Pituitary failure

3. Which of the following is the most likely diagnosis?

- ❑ A Myotonic dystrophy
- ❑ B Craniopharyngioma
- ❑ C Kallmann's syndrome
- ❑ D Friedreich's ataxia
- ❑ E Hereditary sensory-motor neuropathy

Data Interpretation 8 (3 marks)

A 17-year-old woman presents with a six month history of headaches, worst in the morning. Clinical examination, including the cranial nerves and visual acuity are normal. Fundoscopy shows no papilloedema. Her body mass index is 27, her only medication is the oral contraceptive pill and vitamin supplements. Lumbar puncture shows:

Opening pressure	29 cm H_2O
Protein	0.4 g/l
Glucose	5.1 mmol/l
Microscopy	3 lymphocytes/mm^3, no red blood cells

1. Which of the following investigations is the most appropriate?

- ❏ A CT scan of brain
- ❏ B Cytospin
- ❏ C Carotid angiography
- ❏ D MR scan of brain
- ❏ E 24-hour blood pressure profile

2. What is the likely diagnosis?

- ❏ A Migraine
- ❏ B Leukaemic meningitis
- ❏ C Cushing's disease
- ❏ D Phaeochromocytoma
- ❏ E Benign intracranial hypertension

Data Interpretation 9 (5 marks)

A 63-year-old woman is brought into Casualty having been found wandering the streets. She is confused and punches the House Officer during venesection. No focal weakness is found, but the tendon reflexes are reduced.

The following results are obtained:

Hb	106 g/l
WCC	3.3 x 10^9/l
Plt	107 x 10^9/l
Na	129 mmol/l
K	4.6 mmol/l
Urea	3.8 mmol/l
Bilirubin	15 μmol/l
Albumin	42 g/l
Gamma-GT	26 U/l
Creatinine kinase	385 U/l
Total cholesterol	7.9 mmol/l

1. What is the most important investigation?

- ❑ A Chest X-ray
- ❑ B Blood film
- ❑ C Thyroid function tests
- ❑ D Urine osmolality
- ❑ E Enhanced CT of brain

2. What combination of pathologies is most likely to explain the results?

- ❑ A Carcinoma of lung with bone marrow invasion
- ❑ B Alcohol abuse and malnutrition
- ❑ C Drug overdose and aplastic anaemia
- ❑ D Carcinoma of stomach and brain metastases
- ❑ E Hypothyroidism and pernicious anaemia

Data Interpretation 10 (6 marks)

A medical consultation is requested from the labour ward where a 26-year-old Greek woman has become confused after a spontaneous abortion at 9 weeks' gestation. She has ataxia, dysarthria and a pyrexia of 38.2 °C.

A CT scan of the brain is normal but the CSF shows the following changes:

Pressure	21 cm H_2O
Colour	Clear
Protein	0.75 g/l
Glucose	2.0 mmol/l (blood glucose 4.1 mmol/l)
Microscopy	83 cells/mm^3, 81% polymorphonuclear cells

1. What is the likely diagnosis?

❑ A Systemic lupus erythematodes
❑ B Viral meningitis
❑ C Embolic brain abscess
❑ D Listeriosis
❑ E Sinus cavernosus thrombosis

2. How is the diagnosis confirmed?

❑ A Blood cultures
❑ B Auto-antibody screen
❑ C Lupus anti-coagulant estimation
❑ D MR scan of brain
❑ E Polymerase chain reaction

3. Which of the following treatments would you recommend?

❑ A iv hydrocortisone
❑ B iv erythromycin
❑ C iv benzylpenicillin
❑ D Warfarin
❑ E Low-molecular weight heparin

Data Interpretation 11 (4 marks)

A 22-year-old woman presents with bilateral foot drop, slowly worsening over the last five years.

The following neuro-physiological results are obtained:

Radial nerve sensory action potential	< 3 microvolt (> 20 microvolt)
Sural nerve sensory action potential	< 1 microvolt (> 15 microvolt)
Median nerve motor conduction velocity	23 m/s (> 50 m/s)
Peroneal nerve motor conduction velocity	15 m/s (> 45 m/s)

1. What is the likely diagnosis?

- ❑ A Friedreich's ataxia
- ❑ B Subacute combined degeneration of the cord
- ❑ C Multiple sclerosis
- ❑ D Hereditary sensory-motor neuropathy
- ❑ E Tabes dorsalis

2. What is fundoscopy likely to demonstrate?

- ❑ A Normal fundi
- ❑ B Roth spots
- ❑ C Angioid streaks
- ❑ D Papilloedema
- ❑ E Optic atrophy

Data Interpretation 12 (6 marks)

A middle-aged vagrant woman is admitted to the ward after having fallen down the stairs in the local train station.

A CT scan shows a small right chronic subdural haematoma. Three days later she becomes confused with worsening ataxia and horizontal nystagmus in both eyes.
The following results are obtained:

Hb	137 g/l
MCV	102 fl
WCC	9.8×10^9/l (normal differential)
Prothrombin time	16.9 seconds

A lumbar puncture shows normal results.

1. What is the likely diagnosis?

❑ A Subarachnoid haemorrhage
❑ B Extradural haematoma
❑ C Hepatic encephalopathy
❑ D Central pontine myelinolysis
❑ E Wernicke's syndrome

2. What treatment is indicated?

❑ A iv nimodipine
❑ B Surgical decompression
❑ C iv thiamine
❑ D Oral lactulose
❑ E iv glucose

3. What other measures should be considered?

❑ A Fresh frozen plasma
❑ B Oral chlordiazepoxide
❑ C im vitamin B_{12}
❑ D iv hypertonic saline
❑ E im vitamin K

Data Interpretation 13 (4 marks)

A 46-year-old woman has the following neurology:

Wasting of the small muscles of the hands, reduced bicep reflexes and multiple scars and burns over both hands. Sensation to soft touch and vibration is preserved. Fasciculations are seen within the tongue and both legs show increased tone and brisk reflexes.

1. Which of the following diagnoses explains the findings?

❑ A Rheumatoid arthritis
❑ B Syringobulbia
❑ C Motor neurone disease
❑ D Multiple sclerosis
❑ E Cervical spondylosis

2. Which of the following investigations is indicated?

❑ A ESR
❑ B Nerve conduction studies
❑ C Flexion views of cervical spine
❑ D MR scan of cervical spine
❑ E MR scan of brain

Data Interpretation 14 (5 marks)

A 28-year-old woman with difficulties walking is admitted for investigation. The House Officer notices abnormal pupillary reflexes.

	Direct light reaction	**Consensual light reaction**
Right pupil	Absent	Present
Left pupil	Present	Absent

Both eyes show normal reflex on accommodation.

1. What abnormality is consistent with these findings?

❑ A Left optic neuritis
❑ B Right optic atrophy
❑ C Left retinal phakoma
❑ D Right Holmes-Adie pupil
❑ E Left optic glioma

2. What is the likely underlying diagnosis?

❑ A Neurosyphilis
❑ B Neurofibromatosis Type II
❑ C Tuberose sclerosis
❑ D Tobacco amblyopia
❑ E Multiple sclerosis

RESPIRATORY MEDICINE QUESTIONS: CASE HISTORIES

For 'best-of-five' questions candidates must select one answer only, by putting a cross in the appropriate box.

Case History 1 (9 marks)

A 61-year-old housewife is referred by her GP following an 18-month history of slowly worsening shortness of breath on exercise. She was well until six months ago when she started to find it difficult helping her husband with the family-run plumbing business. She smokes 10 cigarettes per day, but is on no regular medication. Her 32-year-old son keeps racing pigeons in the garden, and the couple own two cats.

On examination there is finger clubbing and bilateral fine inspiratory crackles are heard at both lung bases. Examination of heart and abdomen is normal.

A chest X-ray shows lateral pleural thickening in both mid-zones and a small left pleural effusion.

Investigations show:

Hb	138 g/l
WCC	5.9 x 10^9/l (normal differential)
Plt	179 x 10^9/l
ESR	23 mm/hr
U&E's	Normal

Arterial blood gases (on air):	
pH	7.36
pO_2	8.3 kPa (62 mmHg)
pCO_2	4.1 kPa (31 mmHg)
Bicarbonate	21 mmol/l

FEV_1	1.9 l (2.0–3.3 l)
FVC	2.4 l (2.8–4.5 l)
FEV_1/FVC	79%

1. **What is the correct description of her biochemical state?**

- ❑ A Respiratory alkalosis
- ❑ B Metabolic alkalosis
- ❑ C Mixed respiratory and metabolic alkalosis
- ❑ D Compensated respiratory alkalosis
- ❑ E Compensated metabolic acidosis

2. Which of the following investigations is indicated?

- ❑ A Estimation of transfer factor
- ❑ B Auto-antibody screen
- ❑ C High-resolution CT scan
- ❑ D Bronchoscopy and alveolar lavage
- ❑ E Transbronchial lung biopsy

3. What is the likely diagnosis?

- ❑ A Cryptogenic fibrosing alveolitis
- ❑ B Rheumatoid lung
- ❑ C Sarcoidosis
- ❑ D Chronic extrinsic allergic alveolitis
- ❑ E Asbestosis

Two years later she is referred back to clinic with a deterioration of her symptoms, and the following results are obtained:

FEV_1	1.7 l
FVC	2.0 l
FEV_1/FVC	85%
Transfer factor (DLCO)	59%
Transfer coefficient (KCO)	98%

4. What complication has arisen?

- ❑ A Adeno-carcinoma
- ❑ B Tuberculosis
- ❑ C Pleural encasement
- ❑ D Bronchiectasis
- ❑ E Bullous emphysema

Case History 2 (9 marks)

A 36-year-old travelling business man presents with dyspnoea after returning from a trip to the Far East. He has previously been fit and well, but on closer questioning admits to a four-month history of malaise.

On examination he is pale and some small lymph nodes are palpable in the neck. There is hyper-resonant percussion of the right lung apex, clinical examination is otherwise unremarkable. Respiratory rate is 24/min, BP 120/70 mmHg, pulse 108/min, regular. He has an axillary temperature of 38.4 °C.

Investigations show:

Hb	119 g/l
WCC	3.3×10^9/l
Plt	108×10^9/l
Na	136 mmol/l
K	4.1 mmol/l
Urea	10.1 mmol/l
Creatinine	108 µmol/l
Arterial blood gases (room air):	
pH	7.39
pO_2	9.0 kPa (68 mmHg)
pCO_2	3.9 kPa (29 mmHg)

Chest X-ray: Small right apical pneumothorax of 5–10%, no consolidation

1. **What is the likely precipitating cause for the acute presentation?**
2. **What is the likely underlying diagnosis?**
3. **Suggest two further investigations.**
4. **What is the immediate treatment?**

Case History 3 (6 marks)

A 48-year-old farmer is admitted with an episode of haemoptysis. He has had no previous episodes, but has felt unwell with malaise and headaches for the preceding seven weeks. He has lost 3 kg in weight.

On examination he is pyrexial at 37.8 °C. Respiratory rate 22/min, right-sided basal crackles.
Examination of cardiovascular system and abdomen is normal. There is mild proptosis of the left eye, which is tender to palpation. There is minimal diplopia on upward gaze.

Investigations show:

Hb	121 g/l
WCC	7.8 x 10^9/l
Differential: 58% neutrophils, 31% lymphocytes, 2% monocytes	
Plt	468 x 10^9/l
MCV	84 fl
ESR	76 mm/hr
Na	138 mmol/l
K	5.2 mmol/l
Urea	13.3 mmol/l
Creatinine	197 µmol/l
Dipstix urine	Protein ++, Blood ++, Bilirubin -

Chest X-ray: Several ill-defined nodules present in both lungs.

1. What is the likely diagnosis?

- ❑ A Wegener's granulomatosis
- ❑ B Pan-arteritis nodosa
- ❑ C Non-Hodgkin's lymphoma
- ❑ D Goodpasture's syndrome
- ❑ E Extrinsic allergic alveolitis

2. Which of the following is likely to be least useful?

- ❑ A ENT referral
- ❑ B Renal biopsy
- ❑ C Lateral chest X-ray
- ❑ D Auto-antibodies
- ❑ E Serum precipitins

3. What treatment would you recommend?

- ❑ A iv methylprednisolone
- ❑ B iv cyclophosphamide
- ❑ C Radiotherapy
- ❑ D Exposure prophylaxis
- ❑ E Methotrexate

Case History 4 (7 marks)

A 41-year-old Cuban teacher presents with tiredness and three episodes of night sweats. She has lost 2.5 kg in weight over the last three months. She describes an irritating dryness in her throat and dry cough, which has plagued her for the best part of six weeks. In addition, she has recently developed intermittent painful knees and wrists. She had a termination of pregnancy six months earlier and her symptoms seem to have followed on from this. There is no past medical history of note, and her only medication is temazepam for insomnia.

On examination she looks well, no anaemia or jaundice and no evidence of finger clubbing. BP 145/85 mmHg, pulse 56/min, regular, no heart murmurs. One or two lymph nodes are palpated in the axillae, no organomegaly is present in the abdomen. Normal neurological examination.

The following blood results are obtained:

Hb	113 g/l
WCC	6.2 x 10^9/l (normal differential)
Plt	193 x 10^9/l
ESR	59 mm/hr
Na	141 mmol/l
K	4.4 mmol/l
Urea	9.2 mmol/l
Creatinine	112 µmol/l
Albumin	33 g/l
Calcium	2.85 mmol/l
Phosphate	1.3 mmol/l
FEV_1	1.7 l (predicted 2.4–3.7 l)
FVC	2.2 l (predicted 4.0–5.2 l)
TLC	4.8 l (predicted 5.7–7.6 l)

Chest X-ray: Mediastinal widening, clear lungs, normal heart
ECG: Axis -40°, PR 0.25 s, QRS 0.14 s, right bundle branch block, no evidence of ischaemia

1. **Suggest three further investigations.**
2. **What is the complete diagnosis?**
3. **Suggest two important steps in the management.**

Case History 5 (8 marks)

A 59-year-old Turkish blacksmith presents with increasing episodes of haemoptysis. He smokes 25 cigarettes a day and gives a long-standing history of cough, producing sputum on most days first thing in the morning. Initially he only produced small amounts of blood-stained sputum but, over the last two weeks, coughed up a cupful of blood on three occasions.

On examination he is not cyanosed. He has a barrel-shaped chest and there is early finger clubbing. Respiratory rate 20/min. There are crackles at the right base which improve after coughing, no wheeze is heard.
There is a slight right ventricular heave and a pronounced second heart sound, but no cardiac murmurs are heard. BP 160/95 mmHg, pulse 88/min, regular.
The liver edge is palpable 5 cm under the costal margin, spleen or kidneys cannot be palpated.

Blood samples reveal the following results:

Hb	131 g/l
WCC	8.6×10^9/l
Differential: 76% neutrophils, 20% lymphocytes, 3% eosinophils	
Plt	268×10^9/l
ESR	16 mm/hr
U&E's	Normal
FEV_1	2.0 l (predicted 2.4–3.5 l)
FVC	3.2 l (predicted 3.4–4.9 l)
FEV_1/FVC	63%

Chest X-ray: Overinflated lungs, right apical consolidation containing calcification and some air
Bronchoscopy shows no abnormality, bronchial washings are negative for acid-fast bacilli. Cytology shows no evidence of malignancy.

1. What is the likely cause for the patient's symptoms?

- ❑ A Adeno-carcinoma
- ❑ B Pan-arteritis nodosa
- ❑ C Squamous cell carcinoma
- ❑ D Aspergilloma
- ❑ E Histoplasmosis

2. How is the diagnosis confirmed?

- ❑ A Transbronchial lung biopsy
- ❑ B Trans-thoracic lung biopsy
- ❑ C CT scan
- ❑ D Auto-antibody screen
- ❑ E Fungal serology

3. What is the background pulmonary pathology?

- ❑ A Emphysema
- ❑ B Bronchiectasis
- ❑ C Cryptogenic fibrosing alveolitis
- ❑ D Pneumoconiosis
- ❑ E Chronic extrinsic allergic alveolitis

4. What is the treatment of choice?

- ❑ A Direct injection of antibiotics
- ❑ B iv antibiotics
- ❑ C Radiotherapy
- ❑ D Surgery
- ❑ E Steroids

Case History 6 (7 marks)

A 20-year-old man is referred to the chest clinic for investigation of recurrent lower respiratory tract infection. He has been on repeated courses of antibiotics over the last year, but he is still producing yellow sputum most mornings. He can no longer manage to climb the three flights of stairs to his flat in one go, and he has lost 5 kg in weight over the last year.

On examination he is pale but not clubbed. Respiratory rate 22/min, auscultation reveals bilateral early inspiratory crackles and a moderate wheeze. Examination of cardiovascular system and abdomen are unremarkable.

Investigations show:

Hb	138 g/l
WCC	10.3 x 10^9/l (89% neutrophils)
Plt	385 x 10^9/l
ESR	32 mm/hr
Na	136 mmol/l
K	4.1 mmol/l
Urea	8.8 mmol/l
Creatinine	101 μmol/l

Bronchoscopy: Purulent secretions in both lower lobes, no endo-bronchial lesions

ECG: Sinus rhythm 88 bpm, QRS axis +145°, low voltage in lateral chest leads

Sweat Na content 21 mmol/l (20–40 mmol/l)

1. Which of the following is the most useful investigation?

❑ A Blood culture
❑ B Sputum culture
❑ C Chromosomal analysis
❑ D α_1-anti-trypsin levels
❑ E Chest X-ray

2. What is the likely diagnosis?

- ❑ A Cystic fibrosis
- ❑ B Post-infective bronchiectasis
- ❑ C α_1-anti-trypsin deficiency
- ❑ D Kartagener's syndrome
- ❑ E Macleod's syndrome (Swyer-James syndrome)

3. What is the likelihood of his son developing the same condition?

- ❑ A 0%
- ❑ B 25%
- ❑ C 50%
- ❑ D 66%
- ❑ E 100%

Case History 7 (7 marks)

A 64-year-old bachelor presents to the Accident & Emergency Department with severe epigastric pain and nausea and vomiting of three day duration. This was preceded by several weeks of malaise and increasing difficulties getting out of his armchair. He smokes 15 cigarettes per day and has a chronic, dry cough.

On examination he is cachectic with increased skin turgor. The chest is clear. BP 110/70 mmHg with a postural drop of 15 mmHg. No organomegaly. There is bilateral gynaecomastia.

Blood results show:

Hb	108 g/l
WCC	5.6 x 10^9/l (normal differential)
Plt	217 x 10^9/l
MCV	76 fl
ESR	38 mm/hr
Na	144 mmol/l
K	3.2 mmol/l
Urea	16.9 mmol/l
Creatinine	168 μmol/l
Bilirubin	21 U/l
Alkaline phosphatase	428 U/l
ALT	29 U/l
AST	35 U/l
Albumin	33 g/l
Total protein	59 g/l
Calcium	2.95 mmol/l
Radio-isotope bone scan	Generalised increased activity, no focal hot-spots
Bone barrow biopsy	Active erythropoiesis, normal granulopoiesis, 7% plasma cells

1. Which of the following investigations would be the most helpful?

- ❑ A Skeletal survey
- ❑ B Serum phosphate
- ❑ C Ultrasound of liver
- ❑ D Urinary hydroxyproline
- ❑ E Hand X-ray

2. What is the underlying diagnosis?

- ❑ A Squamous cell carcinoma of the lung
- ❑ B Multiple myeloma
- ❑ C Sarcomatous change in Paget's disease
- ❑ D Small cell carcinoma of the lung
- ❑ E Metastasised carcinoma of the colon

3. What is your further management?

- ❑ A iv hydrocortisone and CT scan of chest
- ❑ B iv diphosphonates and serum electrophoresis
- ❑ C iv saline and barium enema
- ❑ D Rectal ion-exchange resins and neck ultrasound
- ❑ E Forced diuresis and chest X-ray

Case History 8 (7 marks)

A 16-year-old girl under investigation for polyuria presents with acute dyspnoea. She had a previous episode six months earlier which had resolved spontaneously. On examination she looks well but distressed. Respiratory rate 28/min. Percussion note in the left upper thorax is hyper-resonant and the breath sounds are reduced. Examination of the abdomen is unremarkable. There is an ejection systolic murmur heard over the aorta, blood pressure 105/65 mmHg, pulse 104/min, regular.

An urgent chest X-ray shows a large, left-sided pneumothorax with early mediastinal shift. In addition there are bilateral interstitial abnormalities with some nodules and multiple cysts.

1. Which of the following diagnoses is least likely?

- ❑ A Tuberose sclerosis
- ❑ B Neurofibromatosis
- ❑ C Eosinophilic granuloma
- ❑ D Sarcoidosis
- ❑ E Lymphangio-leiomyomatosis

A small chest drain is inserted in the X-ray Department and the patient's symptoms are relieved.

Investigations show the following results:

Na	141 mmol/l
K	4.0 mmol/l
Urea	11.0 mmol/l
Creatinine	129 μmol/l
Glucose	4.0 mmol/l
Liver function tests	Normal

Arterial blood gases after drainage of pneumothorax (room air):

pH	7.39
pO_2	9.2 kPa (69 mmHg)
pCO_2	4.3 kPa (29 mmHg)
Bicarbonate	21 mmol/l

2. Which of the following investigations are indicated?

- ❑ A Sputum microscopy and lung function tests
- ❑ B CT thorax and renal biopsy
- ❑ C Lung biopsy and early morning urine sampling
- ❑ D Kveim test and MR brain
- ❑ E Skull X-ray and urine osmolality

3. What complication has probably arisen?

- ❑ A Thalamic dysfunction
- ❑ B Nephrogenic diabetes insipidus
- ❑ C Central diabetes insipidus
- ❑ D Bronchiectasis
- ❑ E Renal tubular acidosis Type II

Case History 9 (5 marks)

A 27-year-old woman presents with a three-day history of painful swallowing and sore throat. Over the last 24-hours she has become breathless on exercise and she has noticed her breathing becoming noisy. She has been given amoxicillin by her GP, her only other medication is the oral contraceptive pill. She has suffered from asthma up to the age of 17 and there is a family history of asthma.

On examination she is anxious and sweating. Respiratory rate 28/min, temperature 38.3 °C. Normal appearances of mouth and fauces. Breath sounds are normal on auscultation, but there is an audible loud inspiratory wheeze. Several lymph nodes are palpable in the anterior cervical triangle. No organomegaly is present in the abdomen.

Investigations reveal:

Hb — 136 g/l
WCC — 16.2×10^9/l
Differential: 77% granulocytes, 15% lymphocytes, 6% monocytes
Plt — 371×10^9/l
ESR — 51 mm/hr

U&E's — Normal

Peak expiratory flow rate — 385 l/min (predicted 440–600 l/min)

Arterial blood gases on air:

pH	7.52
pO_2	11.6 kPa (87 mmHg)
pCO_2	3.5 kPa (26 mmHg)
Bicarbonate	23 mmol/l

Chest radiograph: Overinflated lungs without consolidation

1. What is the most likely diagnosis?

- ❑ A Acute epiglottitis
- ❑ B Hereditary angioedema
- ❑ C Infective exacerbation of asthma
- ❑ D Whooping cough
- ❑ E Acute laryngitis (croup)

2. Which of the following is the most appropriate management?

- ❑ A Urgent ENT referral and intubation
- ❑ B Inhaled salbutamol and iv hydrocortisone
- ❑ C im adrenaline and iv midazolam
- ❑ D iv aminophylline and tracheostomy
- ❑ E iv benzylpenicillin and sc salbutamol

Case History 10 (6 marks)

A 53-year-old steel-worker is referred with malaise, dry cough and exercise-induced dyspnoea. He smokes 20 cigarettes/day but stopped drinking alcohol eight months ago after being told by his GP that he was damaging his liver. One year ago he suffered a severe episode of pyelonephritis which was treated with nitrofurantoin due to a penicillin allergy.

On examination he is clubbed with palmar erythema. Inspiratory crackles are present in both lungs. Respiratory rate 24/min, BP 170/90 mmHg, pulse 92/min, regular. In the abdomen there is 4 cm tender, smooth hepatomegaly, no splenomegaly or lymphadenopathy.

Investigations show:

Hb	151g/l
WCC	5.9 x 10^9/l

Differential: 61% granulocytes, 33% lymphocytes, 3% monocytes

Plt	347 x 10^9/l
ESR	32 mm/hr

Na	142 mmol/l
K	3.8 mmol/l
Urea	9.1 mmol/l
Creatinine	137 μmol/l
Albumin	39 g/l
Total protein	99 g/l
Bilirubin	57 U/l
AST	320 U/l
ALT	270 U/l

A liver biopsy shows areas of piecemeal necrosis.
A high resolution CT scan shows reduced lung volumes, septal thickening and multiple areas of ground-glass change.

Pulmonary function tests reveal:

TLC	3.8 l (predicted 5.7–7.5 l)
FEV_1/FVC	91%

1. Which of the following investigations would be most helpful?

- ❑ A Transbronchial lung biopsy
- ❑ B Auto-antibody screen
- ❑ C Chest X-ray
- ❑ D Lupus anti-coagulant
- ❑ E CO transfer coefficient (KCO)

2. What is the likely respiratory diagnosis?

- ❑ A Occupational asthma
- ❑ B Hypersensitivity pneumonitis
- ❑ C Extrinsic allergic alveolitis
- ❑ D Systemic lupus erythematodes
- ❑ E Cryptogenic fibrosing alveolitis

3. What is the pathology affecting the liver?

- ❑ A Auto-immune chronic active hepatitis
- ❑ B Sclerosing cholangitis
- ❑ C Primary biliary cirrhosis
- ❑ D Heavy metal poisoning
- ❑ E Viral hepatitis

Case History 11 (6 marks)

A 69-year-old Haematology patient is admitted with pleuritic chest pain and a one week history of increasing cough and shortness of breath. Her only current medication is α-interferon.

On examination the patient is tachypnoeic at rest. Temperature 37.9 °C (axilla), BP 115/70 mmHg, pulse 104/min, regular. Examinations of chest and cardiovascular system are normal. There is no lymphadenopathy.

The following results are obtained:

Hb	68 g/l
WCC	25.2 x 10^9/l

Differential: 39% neutrophils, 15% promyelocytes, 23% myeloblasts, 12% lymphocytes, 8% monocytes, 2% eosinophils.

Plt	107 x 10^9/l
ESR	48 mm/hr

U&E's	Normal
Pulse oximetry	93% O_2 saturation on air

Chest X-ray: cavitating left upper lobe pneumonia

1. **What do the blood results indicate?**

❑ A Chronic myeloid leukaemia in blast crisis
❑ B Chronic myelo-monocytic leukaemia
❑ C Acute myeloid leukaemia
❑ D Myelodysplasia
❑ E Leukaemoid reaction

2. **Which of the following is the least likely cause for the respiratory symptoms?**

❑ A Staphylococcal pneumonia
❑ B Tuberculosis
❑ C Cytomegaly virus
❑ D Mycobacterium avium intracellularae
❑ E Klebsiella pneumonia

3. What management would you recommend?

- ❑ A iv amphotericin B and bronchoscopy
- ❑ B Isolation and sputum examination
- ❑ C iv co-trimoxazole and chemotherapy
- ❑ D Intensive care and high-dose oxygen
- ❑ E iv ganciclovir and transfusion

Case History 12 (5 marks)

A 41-year-old flight attendant is referred with intermittent cough and haemoptysis. She also describes intermittent episodes of wheeze, dyspnoea and palpitations. She has otherwise been well with the occasional episode of diarrhoea which she has put down to the frequent travelling. Her symptoms had been investigated 18 months earlier, but a blood test and a chest X-ray had shown normal results. She is on no regular medication and has had all the required vaccines.

On examination she looks wells, clinical examination is normal except for a dull percussion note at the left lung base associated with some reduced breath sounds.

Investigations show:

Hb	141 g/l
WCC	6.5 x 10^9/l (normal differential)
Plt	241 x 10^9/l
ESR	12 mm/hr
Prothrombin time	14 seconds (control 12–14)
U&E's	Normal

Chest X-ray: Partial collapse of left lower lobe, no adenopathy

Arterial blood gases (on air):

pH	7.38
pO_2	12.7 kPa (95 mmHg)
pCO_2	5.5 kPa (41 mmHg)
O_2 sat.	99%

1. **What examination would you recommend?**
2. **What is the likely diagnosis?**

RESPIRATORY MEDICINE QUESTIONS: DATA INTERPRETATIONS

For 'best-of-five' questions candidates must select one answer only, by putting a cross in the appropriate box.

Data Interpretation 1 (4 marks)

An obese 43-year-old woman complains of morning headaches and malaise.

The following results are obtained:

Hb	154 g/l
MCV	101 fl
WCC	6.2×10^9/l (normal differential)

Arterial blood gases (on air):

pO_2	10.4 kPa (78 mmHg)
pCO_2	5.6 kPa (42 mmHg)
Total cholesterol	6.2 mmol/l

1. What is the likely cause for her symptoms?

- ❑ A Type I respiratory failure
- ❑ B Sleep apnoea
- ❑ C Type II respiratory failure
- ❑ D Nocturnal asthma
- ❑ E Diaphragmatic weakness

2. What underlying cause has to be considered?

- ❑ A Cushing's disease
- ❑ B Pernicious anaemia
- ❑ C Cerebral-vascular disease
- ❑ D Cushing's syndrome
- ❑ E Hypothyroidism

Data Interpretation 2 (4 marks)

A 45-year-old man with chronic back pain is found to have an early diastolic murmur. Chest X-ray shows apical interstitial shadowing with a small cavity on the right.

Pulmonary function tests reveal:

FEV_1	2.0 l (predicted 2.1–3.1)
FVC	2.4 l (predicted 3.0–4.4)
TLC	4.8 (predicted 5.0–7.5)
Transfer factor (DLCO)	92%
Transfer coefficient (KCO)	105%

1. **What type of defect is indicated by the results?**
2. **What is the likely diagnosis?**

Data Interpretation 3 (4 marks)

A 64-year-old publican presents with a three-week history of lethargy and coughing up blood-stained sputum. Chest X-ray shows an area of consolidation in the right mid-zone.

Blood results reveal:

Na	136 mmol/l
K	5.4 mmol/l
Urea	29 mmol/l
Creatinine	428 µmol/l

Arterial blood gases (air):

pH	7.29
pO_2	8.8 kPa (66 mmHg)
pCO_2	4.8 kPa (36 mmHg)
Bicarbonate	16 mmol/l

1. Which of the following is the least likely diagnosis?

❑ A Bronchial carcinoma
❑ B Pan-arteritis nodosa
❑ C Goodpasture's syndrome
❑ D Allergic broncho-pulmonary aspergillosis
❑ E Mycoplasma pneumonia

2. Which of the following investigations is least likely to be helpful?

❑ A Sputum microscopy and culture
❑ B Lung biopsy
❑ C CT thorax
❑ D Renal biopsy
❑ E Blood film

Data Interpretation 4 (2 marks)

A 43-year-old non-smoking veterinarian presents with an unproductive cough, worse at night.

Investigations show:

FEV_1	2.4 l (predicted 3.0–4.5)
FVC	3.8 l (predicted 3.9–5.9)
FEV_1/FVC	63%
PEFR	520 l/min (predicted 560–620 l/min)

Methacholine provocation test:
20% fall in FEV_1 is provoked by concentration of 1 mg/ml
(normal > 4 mg/ml)

1. **What diagnosis is suggested by these results?**

- ❑ A Tracheo-malacia
- ❑ B Occupational asthma
- ❑ C Relapsing polychondritis
- ❑ D Hyper-reactive bronchial system
- ❑ E Thyroid enlargement

Data Interpretation 5 (4 marks)

A patient in her twenties is admitted unconscious to the A&E Department. She is tachycardic and tachypnoeic, but haemodynamically stable.

The following results are obtained:

Na	144 mmol/l
K	6.0 mmol/l
Urea	13.6 mmol/l
Chloride	101 mmol/l
Glucose	4.3 mmol/l

Arterial blood gases (room air):

pH	6.96
pO_2	14.1 kPa (106 mmHg)
pCO_2	1.9 kPa (14 mmHg)
Bicarbonate	9 mmol/l

1. **What is the metabolic abnormality?**
2. **What is the likely cause?**

Data Interpretation 6 (4 marks)

A 75-year-old woman presents with a six-week history of malaise and weakness. There is hepatosplenomegaly and a pleural effusion.

Hb 108 g/l
WCC 44 x 10^9/l
Differential: 94% lymphocytes, 2% neutrophils, 2% eosinophils
Plt 93 x 10^9/l
ESR > 120 mm/hr

A pleural tap shows the following results:

Protein 48 g/l
Glucose 1.8 mmol/l
Microscopy: Lymphocytes +++, no bacteria on Gram stain, no AAFB seen

1. What is your next investigation?

❑ A Silver stain of pleural fluid
❑ B Serial blood cultures
❑ C Sputum culture and microscopy
❑ D Bone marrow biopsy
❑ E Abdominal ultrasound scan

2. What is the diagnosis?

❑ A Non-Hodgkin's lymphoma
❑ B Chronic lymphocytic leukaemia
❑ C TB empyema
❑ D Histoplasmosis
❑ E Sézary syndrome

Data Interpretation 7 (4 marks)

A 23-year-old woman presents with acute onset of breathlessness. She is nine weeks pregnant and has always been well. Respiratory rate 28/min, pulse 92/min regular, BP 155/70 mmHg.

FBC	Normal

Arterial blood gases (room air) reveal:

pH	7.55
pO_2	13.8 kPa (99 mmHg)
pCO_2	7.5 kPa (21 mmHg)
Bicarbonate	20 mmol/l

1. What would be your management?

- ❑ A iv heparin
- ❑ B Chest X-ray
- ❑ C iv midazolam
- ❑ D Re-breathing from paper bag
- ❑ E Administration of 40% O_2

2. What is the likely diagnosis?

- ❑ A Hyperventilation
- ❑ B Pulmonary embolus
- ❑ C Pneumothorax
- ❑ D Diaphragmatic splinting
- ❑ E Pulmonary oedema

Data Interpretation 8 (5 marks)

A 36-year-old bank manager presents with a 10-day history of productive cough and malaise.

Investigations show:

Hb	92 g/l
RCC	2.6×10^{12}/l
Reticulocytes	4.6%
WCC	9.8×10^{9}/l
Differential: 41% granulocytes, 52% lymphocytes, 4% monocytes	
Plt	381×10^{9}/l
Dipstix urine	Blood +++, Protein +, Glucose -
Chest X-ray: Bilateral patchy basal consolidation	

1. What is the likely diagnosis?

- ❑ A Glucose-6-phosphate dehydrogenase deficiency
- ❑ B Haemolytic uraemic syndrome
- ❑ C Mycoplasma pneumonia
- ❑ D Paroxysmal nocturnal haemoglobinuria
- ❑ E Sickle cell disease

2. Which of the following tests will be positive for haemolysis?

- ❑ A Direct Coombs' test
- ❑ B Indirect Coombs' test
- ❑ C Ham's test (acidic resistance)
- ❑ D Osmotic resistance
- ❑ E Heat resistance at 40 °C

Data Interpretation 9 (4 marks)

A 16-year-old asthmatic patient is admitted with breathlessness. There is only minimal wheeze on auscultation. The patient receives two doses of oxygen-driven nebulised bronchodilators and a subsequent arterial blood sample shows the following results:

pH	7.35
pO_2	8.1 kPa (61 mmHg)
pCO_2	5.7 kPa (43 mmHg)
Chest X-ray	Clear lungs, no pneumothorax

1. **Which of the following would be the most appropriate management?**

❑ A iv hydrocortisone and 60% O_2
❑ B iv aminophylline and 28% O_2
❑ C iv doxapram and 95% O_2
❑ D Nebulised adrenaline on air
❑ E Subcutaneous salbutamol injections and anaesthetic assessment

Data Interpretation 10 (4 marks)

A 32-year-old foundry worker with long-standing mild asthma develops productive cough, fever and wheeze resistant to inhaled salbutamol.

Blood results reveal:

Hb	142 g/l
WCC	9.2×10^9/l

Differential: 61% neutrophils, 23% lymphocytes, 11% eosinophils, 4% monocytes

Plt	217×10^9/l
ESR	59 mm/hr

Three sputum samples and three early morning urines are negative for acid-fast bacilli.

1. **What is the likely diagnosis?**
2. **Suggest two investigations that confirm the diagnosis.**

Data Interpretation 11 (4 marks)

A 23-year-old man with progressive breathlessness shows the following results on lung function tests:

FEV_1	2.0 l
FVC	3.8 l
FEV_1/FVC	53%
TLC	6.1 l (predicted 4.5–5.9 l)
Transfer coefficient (KCO)	73%

1. What do the results suggest?

- ❑ A Emphysema
- ❑ B Small airway obstruction
- ❑ C Bronchiectasis
- ❑ D Fibrosis
- ❑ E Haemorrhage

2. What is the likely diagnosis?

- ❑ A Asthma
- ❑ B Cystic fibrosis
- ❑ C Rheumatoid arthritis
- ❑ D α_1-antitrypsin deficiency
- ❑ E Hereditary haemorrhagic telangiectasia

Data Interpretation 12 (2 marks)

A 21-year-old nurse is admitted for investigation of breathlessness and diplopia. Except for an episode of prolonged diarrhoea three months previously she has always been well. The following results are obtained:

FEV_1	2.1 l (predicted 3.8–4.2)
FVC	2.5 l (predicted 4.2–5.0)

Arterial gases (room air):

pH	7.30
pO_2	9.8 kPa (73.5 mmHg)
pCO_2	6.1 kPa (46 mmHg)

1. Which of the following is the most likely diagnosis?

❑ A Phrenic nerve palsy
❑ B Guillain-Barré syndrome
❑ C Myasthenia gravis
❑ D Multiple sclerosis
❑ E Organophosphate poisoning

Data Interpretation 13 (5 marks)

A 68-year-old woman presents with polyarthritis, low-grade fever and exercise-induced dyspnoea.

The following results are obtained:

Hb	103 g/l
WCC	7.1×10^9/l (normal differential)
Plt	528×10^9/l
CRP	43 mg/l (< 10 mg/l)

FEV_1/FVC	58%
Total lung capacity	5.0 l (predicted 4–5.2 l)
Residual capacity	0.7 l (predicted 0.5–0.9 l)
Transfer coefficient (KCO)	99%
Pulse oximetry (on air)	99% O_2-saturation

1. What is the likely diagnosis?

- ❑ A Rheumatoid arthritis
- ❑ B Systemic sclerosis
- ❑ C Relapsing polychondritis
- ❑ D Extrinsic allergic alveolitis
- ❑ E Churg-Strauss syndrome

2. What would you expect to find on the chest X-ray?

- ❑ A Normal appearances
- ❑ B Basal fibrosis
- ❑ C Apical fibrosis
- ❑ D Pleural effusion
- ❑ E Alveolar shadowing

Data Interpretation 14 (3 marks)

A 55-year-old smoker presents with abdominal pain and confusion. Biopsy shows a small vessel necrotizing vasculitis.

A chest X-ray shows bilateral lower zone alveolar shadowing and small pleural effusions.

Investigations show:

Na	125 mmol/l
K	3.9 mmol/l
Urea	10.1 mmol/l
Creatinine	162 µmol/l
Bilirubin	28 µmol/l
AST	61 U/l
Albumin	29 g/l
Sputum: Negative Gram stain, Negative culture	
O_2-sat.	93% on air

1. What is your management?

- ❑ A Insertion of central line and 60% O_2 administration
- ❑ B iv diuretics and cardiac enzyme levels
- ❑ C Blood cultures and iv amoxicillin
- ❑ D ECG and iv albumin
- ❑ E Arterial blood gases and iv erythromycin

Data Interpretation 15 (4 marks)

A 36-year-old patient with recurrent nose bleeds presents with haemoptysis and shortness of breath. The following results are obtained:

Hb	119 g/l
MCV	70 fl
ESR	28 mm/hr
FEV_1/ FVC	85%
Transfer coefficient (KCO)	162%
Arterial blood gases (room air):	
pH	7.49
pO_2	9.2 kPa (69 mmHg)
pCO_2	3.6 kPa (27 mmHg)
Bicarbonate	23 mmol/l
Chest X-ray	Right basal consolidation

1. What has precipitated the acute presentation?

- ❑ A Pulmonary embolus
- ❑ B Pulmonary haemorrhage
- ❑ C Aspiration
- ❑ D Pneumothorax
- ❑ E Superinfection

2. What is the likely diagnosis?

- ❑ A Haemophilia
- ❑ B Idiopathic thrombocytopenic purpura
- ❑ C von Willebrand-Jürgen's syndrome
- ❑ D Hereditary haemorrhagic telangiectasia
- ❑ E Wegener's granulomatosis

Data Interpretation 16 (4 marks)

A 43-year-old woman with sero-positive rheumatoid arthritis is prescribed indomethacin for increasing pain in her right hip. Two months later she returns complaining of breathlessness.

Lung function tests in clinic show:

FEV_1	3.0 l (predicted 2.8–3.3 l)
FVC	3.8 l (predicted 3.4–4.3 l)
FEV_1/FVC	79%
PEFR	510 l/min (predicted 490–580 l/min)
O_2-sat.	98% on air

1. **Which of the following investigations is least likely to be helpful?**

- ❑ A Full blood count
- ❑ B Chest X-ray
- ❑ C Arterial blood gases
- ❑ D Biochemical profile
- ❑ E Erythrocyte sedimentation rate

2. **Which of the following is least likely to have produced her symptoms?**

- ❑ A Renal failure
- ❑ B Bronchospasm
- ❑ C Anaemia
- ❑ D Pulmonary fibrosis
- ❑ E Fluid retention

Data Interpretation 17 (4 marks)

A 37-year-old female secretary presents with acute onset of dyspnoea. Clinical examination and a chest radiograph are normal.

Investigations show:

FEV_1	2.7 l (predicted 2.5–3.8 l)
FVC	3.8 l (predicted 3.2–5.9 l)

Arterial blood gases (room air):

pH	7.45
pO_2	9.5 kPa (71 mmHg)
pCO_2	4.1 kPa (31 mmHg)

Ventilation-perfusion scan: two sub-segmental mismatched defects, intermediate probability for embolus.

1. Which of the following is the most appropriate investigation?

- ❑ A CT angiogram
- ❑ B Chest X-ray in expiration
- ❑ C D-dimer levels
- ❑ D Serology for atypical infection
- ❑ E Full blood count

2. What is the likely diagnosis?

- ❑ A Hyperventilation
- ❑ B Pulmonary embolus
- ❑ C Pneumothorax
- ❑ D Mycoplasma infection
- ❑ E Macleod's syndrome

Data Interpretation 18 (3 marks)

A 29-year-old woman with anti-phospholipid syndrome presents with a dry cough and mild wheeze. In the past she had two miscarriages.

The following results are obtained:

Hb	113 g/l
MCV	79 fl
WCC	7.3 x 10^9/l
Differential: 51% neutrophils, 37% lymphocytes, 8% eosinophils	
Plt	258 x 10^9/l
ESR	33 mm/hr
PT	13 sec (11–13 sec)
APTT	58 sec (28–4 sec)
Bleeding time	11 sec (control 6–9 sec)

A chest radiograph shows ill-defined infiltrates in the periphery of both lungs.

1. **What is the likely diagnosis?**

- ❑ A Fungal infection
- ❑ B Loeffler syndrome
- ❑ C Churg-Strauss syndrome
- ❑ D Drug side-effects
- ❑ E Pan-arteritis nodosa

Data Interpretation 19 (4 marks)

A 57-year-old patient presents with dysphagia and breathlessness.

The following results are obtained:

Hb	106 g/l
WCC	5.6 x 10^9/l (normal differential)
Plt	227 x 10^9/l
MCV	73 fl
ESR	21 mm/hr
CRP	4.5 mg/dl (< 10 mg/dl)
FEV_1	3.6 l (predicted 3.4–4.2 l)
FVC	4.0 l (predicted 4.8–5.4 l)
Transfer coefficient (KCO)	87%

Chest X-ray: Interstitial shadowing in both lower zones

1. Which of the following is the most appropriate investigation?

- ❑ A Barium swallow
- ❑ B Auto-antibody screen
- ❑ C Trans-bronchial lung biopsy
- ❑ D Spiral CT thorax
- ❑ E Oesophageal manometry

2. Which of the following diagnoses is unlikely?

- ❑ A Achalasia
- ❑ B Systemic sclerosis
- ❑ C Tylosis
- ❑ D Whipple's disease
- ❑ E Hiatus hernia

Data Interpretation 20 (5 marks)

A 73-year-old man is admitted to hospital with an infective exacerbation of chronic airflow limitation. Investigations show:

Arterial blood gases (on air):

pH	7.31
pO_2	6.5 kPa (49 mmHg)
pCO_2	7.1 kPa (53 mmHg)
Bicarbonate	27 mmol/l

He is treated with nebulisers and transferred to the ward where he deteriorates over the following two hours.

Repeat arterial gases show:

pH	7.23
pO_2	9.8 kPa (74 mmHg)
pCO_2	9.3 kPa (70 mmHg)
Bicarbonate	28 mmol/l

A portable chest X-ray shows extensive right mid-zone consolidation.

1. What is the likely cause for the deterioration?

- ❑ A Aspiration
- ❑ B Septicaemia
- ❑ C Adult respiratory distress syndrome (ARDS)
- ❑ D CO_2 narcosis
- ❑ E O_2 administration

2. What management would you recommend?

- ❑ A iv antibiotics
- ❑ B Insertion of nasogastric tube
- ❑ C Intubation
- ❑ D iv doxapram
- ❑ E High-dose O_2 administration

Data Interpretation 21 (2 marks)

Following a holiday in Mexico, a 41-year-old rock-climber presents with pyrexia, dry cough and polyarthralgia. Erythema nodosum is present on his shins.

Examinations reveal:

Hb	153 g/l
WCC	10.1 x 10^9/l
Differential: 62% neutrophils, 31% lymphocytes, 4% eosinophils	
Plt	309 x 10^9/l
ESR	41 mm/hr

Chest X-ray: Diffuse micro-nodular infiltrates, hilar and mediastinal adenopathy

1. What is the likely diagnosis?

- ❑ A Varicella pneumonia
- ❑ B Acute sarcoidosis
- ❑ C Tuberculosis
- ❑ D Non-Hodgkin's lymphoma
- ❑ E Histoplasmosis

Data Interpretation 22 (5 marks)

A 23-year-old student is admitted unconscious to the A&E Department. A friend indicates that he has been suffering from headaches and malaise for several weeks. He is tachypnoeic, hyper-reflexic and pyrexial but not cyanosed.

Investigations reveal:

Arterial gases (on air):

pH	6.72
pO_2	6.8 kPa (51 mmHg)
pCO_2	2.4 kPa (18 mmHg)
Bicarbonate	23 mmol/l
O_2-sat.	61%

Chest X-ray: Normal

1. What is the likely diagnosis?

- ❑ A Aspirin overdose
- ❑ B Carbon monoxide poisoning
- ❑ C Paracetamol overdose
- ❑ D Methanol poisoning
- ❑ E Ecstasy overdose

2. What is the immediate treatment?

- ❑ A iv acetylcysteine
- ❑ B Exchange transfusion
- ❑ C iv bicarbonate
- ❑ D iv ethanol
- ❑ E Hyperbaric oxygen

Data Interpretation 23 (4 marks)

A 61-year-old woman presents with malaise, weight loss and copious amounts of frothy sputum, worst in the morning.

Investigations show:

Hb	102 g/l
MCV	73 fl
WCC	6.9×10^9/l (normal differential)
Plt	191×10^9/l
Pulse oximetry	94% saturation on air

Chest X-ray: Large area of consolidation in left upper lobe

1. What investigation would you recommend?

- ❑ A Sputum Gram stain and culture
- ❑ B Bronchoscopy and biopsy
- ❑ C Video fluoroscopy
- ❑ D Gastroscopy
- ❑ E High-resolution CT thorax

2. What is the likely diagnosis?

- ❑ A Tracheo-oesophageal fistula
- ❑ B Alveolar cell carcinoma
- ❑ C Bronchiectasis
- ❑ D Cardiac failure
- ❑ E Zenker diverticulum

Data Interpretation 24 (4 marks)

A 47-year-old line manager in a cheese factory presents with worsening breathlessness. Examination reveals a few inspiratory crackles but no other abnormality.

The following results are obtained:

FBC	Normal
PEFR	550 l/min (predicted 590–650 l/min)
FEV_1/FVC	78%
O_2-sat.	95% on air
Transfer coefficient (KCO)	88%

1. What is the likely diagnosis?

- ❑ A Emphysema
- ❑ B Occupational asthma
- ❑ C Extrinsic allergic alveolitis
- ❑ D Chronic bronchitis
- ❑ E Allergic broncho-pulmonary aspergillosis

2. What is his chest X-ray likely to show?

- ❑ A Apical fibrosis
- ❑ B Basal fibrosis
- ❑ C Bullae
- ❑ D Pleural thickening
- ❑ E Bronchiectasis

RHEUMATOLOGY QUESTIONS: CASE HISTORIES

For 'best-of-five' questions candidates must select one answer only, by putting a cross in the appropriate box.

Case History 1 (10 marks)

A 37-year-old man presents to his GP with a painful penile ulcer. A swab is taken for culture and the patient started on oral amoxicillin. 10 days later he is admitted with photophobia and neck stiffness. On examination there is no focal neurology and both plantars are downgoing. Over his right shin several purple, coalescent nodules are seen and he has a pustular rash over his trunk. In addition, he has painful swelling of both knees and the left elbow. Examination of chest and cardiovascular system is unremarkable. Fundoscopy is normal, but both eyes are red with ciliary injection.

The following results are obtained:

Hb	142 g/l
WCC	9.8 x 10^9/l
Differential: 64% neutrophils, 31% lymphocytes, 4% eosinophils	
Plt	476 x 10^9/l
ESR	38 mm/hr
Biochemical profile	Normal
Bilirubin	19 µmol/l
AST	18 U/l
Glucose	5.9 mmol/l

One day later pustules have formed at the venaepuncture sites.

1. Which of the following investigations would you recommend?

❑ A HLA-B27
❑ B Joint aspiration
❑ C CT brain scan
❑ D Blood cultures
❑ E Skin biopsy

A lumbar puncture is performed with the following results:
CSF blood stained, no xanthochromia

Opening pressure	14 cm H_2O
Protein	0.45 g/l
Glucose	3.1 g/l
Microscopy [/mm^3]	18 mononuclear cells
	12 red cells

2. What do these results suggest?

- ❑ A Viral meningitis
- ❑ B Bacterial meningitis
- ❑ C Subarachnoid haemorrhage
- ❑ D Traumatic tap
- ❑ E Brain abscess

3. What is the likely diagnosis?

- ❑ A Gonorrhoea
- ❑ B Reiter's syndrome
- ❑ C Behçet's disease
- ❑ D Lymphogranuloma venereum
- ❑ E Syphilis

4. What treatment would you recommend?

- ❑ A iv gentamicin
- ❑ B Systemic steroids
- ❑ C im penicillin
- ❑ D Oral doxycycline
- ❑ E iv cyclosporin

After an initial recovery, the patient becomes severely obtunded with a Glasgow Coma Scale of 5/15. A CT scan shows bilateral deep white matter haemorrhage.

5. What complication has occurred?

- ❑ A Superior sagittal sinus thrombosis
- ❑ B Cerebral vasculitis
- ❑ C Disseminated intravascular coagulation
- ❑ D Auto-immune thrombocytopenia
- ❑ E Over-anticoagulation

Case History 2 (7 marks)

A 61-year-old woman is referred for investigation with a three-month history of malaise and difficulties climbing the stairs to her first floor flat. She also complains of difficulties swallowing, particularly with solids which cause retro-sternal pain. On examination she is pale, no lymph-adenopathy. CNS and respiratory system are unremarkable. The liver edge is firm and irregular, the spleen is not palpable and there is no adenopathy.

The following results are obtained:

Hb	98 g/l
MCV	69 fl
WCC	5.8 x 10^9/l
Plt	219 x 10^9/l
ESR	66 mm/hr
MCHC	25 g/dl
U&E's	Normal
Bilirubin	22μmol/l
AST	520 U/l
Gamma GT	29 U/l
Alkaline phosphatase	112 U/l
Anti-nuclear antibodies	1:1024

A gastroscopy shows normal oesophagus and stomach.

1. Which of the following investigations would you perform next?

- ❑ A Temporal artery biopsy
- ❑ B Creatinine kinase
- ❑ C Fundoscopy
- ❑ D Anti-ds-DNA-antibodies
- ❑ E Acetylcholine-receptor antibodies

An EMG shows evidence of fibrillation and polyphasic bursts.

2. What is the diagnosis?

- ❑ A Polymyalgia rheumatica
- ❑ B Motor neurone disease
- ❑ C Myasthenia gravis
- ❑ D Systemic lupus erythematodes
- ❑ E Polymyositis

3. What further investigation would you perform?

- ❑ A Muscle biopsy
- ❑ B Barium enema
- ❑ C Tensilon test
- ❑ D Electrocardiogram
- ❑ E Oesophageal manometry

Case History 3 (9 marks)

A 34-year-old prostitute is referred from the Casualty Department with a left-sided weakness affecting the arm more than the leg. This had developed overnight, but had been preceded by two previous episodes of weakness in the left, non-dominant hand. Prior to this she had always been well and apart from the oral contraceptive pill was on no other medication. She does not drink alcohol, but smokes 10 cigarettes per day.

On examination there is a 3/5 weakness of the left arm and 4/5 weakness of the left leg, the plantar is up-going and non-sustained clonus is present in the left ankle. There is minor impairment of rapid alternating movements and a few beats of nystagmus are present in both eyes on extreme abduction. There is no meningism, on fundoscopy the discs appear normal but some silver-wiring is present on both sides.

BP 170/95 mmHg, pulse 88/min, regular, no heart murmurs on auscultation. The lungs are clear. Axillary temperature 38.3 °C. Examination of the gait reveals a right-sided limp and difficulties walking heel-to-toe.

The following results are obtained:

Hb	100 g/l
MCV	81 fl
WCC	3.9 x 10^9/l
Plt	127 x 10^9/l
MCH	27 pg
Na	130 mmol/l
K	4.9 mmol/l
Creatinine	168 μmol/l
Total protein	76 g/l
Albumin	31 g/l
Bilirubin	17 μmol/l
AST	39 U/l
CRP	8.5 mg/l (< 10 mg/l)
VDRL	Positive 1:512
Urine dipstix	Blood +, Protein +++

1. What is the likely diagnosis?

❑ A Multiple sclerosis
❑ B Neurosyphilis
❑ C Systemic lupus erythematodes
❑ D HIV infection
❑ E Polyarteritis nodosa

2. Which of the following investigations is the most useful?

❑ A Blood and urine cultures
❑ B Lumbar puncture
❑ C CT scan of the brain
❑ D Treponema pallidum haemagglutination tests
❑ E Renal biopsy

Over the following fortnight, the patient makes a slow recovery, however the limp is becoming worse. A plain radiograph shows no abnormality but a bone scan shows increased uptake of radioisotope over the right hip.

3. What is the likely pathology?

❑ A Avascular necrosis
❑ B Septic arthritis
❑ C Neuropathic joint
❑ D Reactive arthritis
❑ E Stress fracture

While awaiting orthopaedic review, the patient develops bilateral ankle swelling and dyspnoea. The percussion note is stony dull at both lung bases.

4. What complication has developed?

❑ A Myocarditis
❑ B Nephrotic syndrome
❑ C Pyelonephritis
❑ D Pericarditis
❑ E Aortic dissection

Case History 4 (8 marks)

A 48-year-old switchboard operator is in long-term follow-up for sero-positive nodular rheumatoid arthritis. She is referred by her GP as an urgency, with a 10 day history of intermittent diplopia.

Her arthritis had flared up eight months previously and she had been successfully started on indomethacin 50 mg/bd and D-penicillamine 500 mg/daily. Blood results at that time were normal. She is also on thyroxine 200 µg following radio-iodine ablation for thyrotoxicosis.
On examination there is only mild synovial swelling in the small joints of the hands. Moderate ulnar deviation is present in the MCP joints.
Neurological examination reveals mild weakness of the upper limbs, more pronounced after exercise, but there is no evidence of wasting or fasciculation. Reflexes are present with reinforcement. Cranial nerves are unremarkable. Some fine end-inspiratory crackles are heard at the lung bases which do not clear with coughing. BP 150/85 mmHg, pulse 76/min, regular, respiratory rate 22/min.

Blood results:

Hb	118 g/l
WCC	5.6 x 10^9/l
Plt	102 x 10^9/l
MCV	79 fl
ESR	16 mm/hr
Na	141 mmol/l
K	3.9 mmol/l
Creatinine	168 µmol/l
Albumin	29 g/l

1. **Which two of the following investigations would be the most useful?**

- ❑ A Chest X-ray and 24 hr creatinine clearance
- ❑ B Rheumatoid factor and bone marrow biopsy
- ❑ C Urinary protein and acetylcholine receptor antibodies
- ❑ D Renal biopsy and auto-antibody screen
- ❑ E High resolution CT chest and histone anti-bodies

2. What is the likely underlying cause for the neurology?

- ❑ A Recurrence of thyrotoxicosis
- ❑ B Myasthenia gravis
- ❑ C Drug-induced lupus
- ❑ D Drug-induced myasthenia
- ❑ E Mono-neuritis multiplex

3. What therapeutic measure would you recommend?

- ❑ A Reduce thyroxine
- ❑ B Stop indomethacin
- ❑ C Stop penicillamine
- ❑ D Introduce steroids
- ❑ E Start pyridostigmine

4. What is the most likely cause for the respiratory signs?

- ❑ A Rheumatoid lung
- ❑ B Chronic aspiration
- ❑ C Drug-induced fibrosis
- ❑ D Cryptogenic fibrosing alveolitis
- ❑ E Invasive aspergillosis

Case History 5 (6 marks)

A 42-year-old Egyptian travel agent presents with an 18-month history of back pain and intermittent arthritis of both knees and elbows. Lately he has also noticed a decrease in exercise tolerance and has had intermittent right-sided pleuritic chest pains. He also gives a history of episodic diarrhoea, but a colonoscopy and small bowel enema performed six months previously showed no abnormalities. He is on no current medication, drinks 25 units of alcohol per week and does not smoke.

Small effusions are present in both knees, examination of the spine reveals a full range of movements, but tenderness over the right sacro-iliac joint. Chest examination shows dullness on percussion at the right base, but no crackles. Cardiovascular system is unremarkable.

The following blood results are obtained:

Hb	105 g/l
WCC	4.8 x 10^9/l
Plt	193 x 10^9/l
MCV	103 fl
MCHC	22 g/dl
ESR	47 mm/hr
Na	139 mmol/l
K	4.2 mmol/l
Urea	5.2 mmol/l
Albumin	31 g/l
Calcium	2.0 mmol/l
Bilirubin	15 µmol/l
Gamma GT	19 U/l

X-rays show a small right-sided pleural effusion and a globular heart. Sclerosis around both SI joints is present, worse on the right.

A radio-labelled white cell scan shows normal appearance of the abdomen, but some increased activity at the pleural surfaces and the mediastinum.

1. What investigation would you recommend?

- ❑ A Joint aspirate
- ❑ B Small bowel biopsy
- ❑ C Pleural aspirate
- ❑ D Gliadin antibodies
- ❑ E Auto-antibody screen

2. What is the likely diagnosis?

- ❑ A Coeliac disease
- ❑ B Crohn's disease
- ❑ C Tropical sprue
- ❑ D Whipple's disease
- ❑ E Familial Mediterranean fever

3. What is the appropriate therapy?

- ❑ A Tetracycline
- ❑ B Mesalazine
- ❑ C Oral steroids
- ❑ D Colchicine
- ❑ E Diclofenac

Case History 6 (6 marks)

A 53-year-old man is referred for investigation of low grade pyrexia and night sweats. He has lost 5 kg in weight over six months. More recently he has become breathless, and has experienced some relief by a salbutamol inhaler. He has a two-year history of angina which is controlled on oral nitrates and aspirin.

On examination there is some tenderness of the wrists and knees, but no active synovitis.

Mild pitting oedema is seen around both ankles, BP 175/100 mmHg, pulse 80/min, regular. Fine crackles are auscultated at the bases and there is a generalised wheeze. Investigations reveal:

Hb	138 g/l
WCC	10.5 x 10^9/l
Differential: 81% granulocytes, 6% eosinophils, 12% lymphocytes	
Plt	482 x 10^9/l
ESR	53 mm/hr
MCV	81 fl
MCH	29 pg

Na	136 mmol/l
K	5.1 mmol/l
Urea	14.2 mmol/l
Creatinine	261 µmol/l
Albumin	36 g/l
LFT's	Normal

1. What is the likely diagnosis?

- ❑ A Panarteritis nodosa
- ❑ B Wegener's granulomatosis
- ❑ C Systemic lupus erythematodes
- ❑ D Pulmonary eosinophilia
- ❑ E Churg-Strauss syndrome

2. How would you confirm the diagnosis?

❑ A Lung biopsy
❑ B Nasal biopsy
❑ C Renal angiogram
❑ D Anti-neutrophil-cytoplasmatic antibodies (ANCA)
❑ E Antibodies to double-stranded DNA

3. What is the most important prognostic factor?

❑ A Degree of renal involvement
❑ B Degree of arterial involvement
❑ C Degree of CNS involvement
❑ D Pattern of auto-antibodies
❑ E CRP levels

Case History 7 (9 marks)

A 13-year-old Chinese boy is referred with a three-week history of intermittent pyrexia and night sweats. He has also been complaining of pain in the right knee and left ankle and he has developed tender nodules over both shins.

His mother complains that, over the last week, he has started to drop things and has broken both teapots. The patient had a previously unremarkable childhood, had all routine vaccinations, but had caught chicken pox eight months previously and scarlet fever two months ago.

On examination he has tender, swollen wrists and elbows but the joints of the lower limbs appear to have settled. Mild erythema nodosum is present. The chest is clear and the abdomen is soft without organomegaly. Examination of the CNS is unremarkable without evidence of cerebellar signs, however some involuntary movements of the right hand are observed. BP 110/55 mmHg, PR 88/min, no murmurs on auscultation.

The following results are obtained:

Hb	106 g/l
WCC	9.8 x 10^9/l (72% neutrophils)
Plt	428 x 10^9/l
CRP	28 mg/dl
Na	136 mmol/l
K	4.1 mmol/l
Urea	5.6 mmol/l
Creatinine	73 μmol/l
LFT's	Normal
Paul Bunnell test	Negative
Rheumatoid factor	Negative
Chest X-ray	Normal
X-rays of hands and feet	No osteoporosis, no erosions

The patient is started on aspirin with a rapid symptomatic improvement.

1. **Suggest two further investigations.**
2. **What is the likely underlying diagnosis?**
3. **What is the cause for the neurological findings?**
4. **What further management has to be considered?**

RHEUMATOLOGY QUESTIONS: DATA INTERPRETATIONS

For 'best-of-five' questions candidates must select one answer only, by putting a cross in the appropriate box.

Data Interpretation 1 (5 marks)

A 32-year-old farmer presents to the Neurology Department with a left-sided facial weakness. Over the previous six weeks he developed aches and pains in muscles and joints and intermittently had to stop working.

On examination, Bell's phenomenon is positive, but he is able to wrinkle his forehead normally.

Hb	119 g/l
WCC	6.1×10^9/l (65% neutrophils)
Plt	375×10^9/l
ESR	58 mm/hr
Biochemical profile	Normal
Auto-antibody screen	Negative

1. What is the likely diagnosis?

❑ A Reiter's syndrome
❑ B Bell's palsy
❑ C Heerfordt syndrome
❑ D Lyme disease
❑ E Behçet's syndrome

2. What investigation is likely to be most useful?

❑ A Chest X-ray
❑ B HLA-B27
❑ C Borrelia serology
❑ D Joint aspirate
❑ E Skin biopsy

Data Interpretation 2 (4 marks)

A 33-year-old Jamaican woman is referred for investigation of heartburn and dysphagia. Gastroscopy is normal, blood results show:

Hb	113 g/l
WCC	6.1×10^9/l
MCV	81 fl
ESR	33 mm/hr
Anti-nuclear antibodies	1:640, speckled pattern
Anti-centromere	1:10
Scl-70	1:160
Anti-Nucleolus	1:160
Anti-ds DNA	1:10
Anti-ENA	1:10

1. What is the likely diagnosis?

- ❑ A Sjögren's syndrome
- ❑ B Limited cutaneous systemic sclerosis (CREST)
- ❑ C Diffuse systemic sclerosis
- ❑ D Systemic lupus erythematodes
- ❑ E Mixed connective tissue disease (Sharp syndrome)

2. What is the next investigation?

- ❑ A Dipstix urine
- ❑ B CRP
- ❑ C Chest X-ray
- ❑ D Blood pressure measurement
- ❑ E MR of oesophagus

Data Interpretation 3 (4 marks)

A 36-year-old man on polychemotherapy for a relapse of Stage III B Hodgkin's disease, presents with increasing shortness of breath. On examination there are bilateral basal crackles and pitting oedema of the lower legs. Palpation of the abdomen reveals hepato-splenomegaly.

Na	132 mmol/l
K	5.1 mmol/l
Urea	13.6 mmol/l
Creatinine	197 μmol/l
Albumin	28 g/l

Chest X-ray: Widened mediastinum, cardiomegaly, interstitial pulmonary oedema

Ultrasound abdomen: Hepato-splenomegaly, large kidneys without evidence of obstruction

1. What is the likely diagnosis?

- ❑ A Renal lymphoma
- ❑ B Membranous glomerulonephritis
- ❑ C Cytostatic-induced cardiomyopathy
- ❑ D Reactive amyloidosis
- ❑ E Renal vein thrombosis

2. What investigation would confirm this?

- ❑ A Echocardiogram
- ❑ B Renal biopsy
- ❑ C MAG-3 renogram
- ❑ D Intravenous urogram
- ❑ E Enhanced CT abdomen

Data Interpretation 4 (5 marks)

A 43-year-old lady with long-standing, severe psoriasis is started on methotrexate 30 mg/week. After 10 days her left knee becomes swollen, hot and painful overnight. The following results are obtained:

Hb	122 g/l
WCC	4.2×10^9/l
Plt	95×10^9/l
ESR	36 mm/hr
U&E's	Normal

Knee X-ray: Small amount of calcification within the articular cartilage, no bone destruction

1. What is the likely diagnosis?

- ❑ A Calcium pyrophosphate deposition
- ❑ B Septic arthritis
- ❑ C Acute gout
- ❑ D Joint haemorrhage
- ❑ E Psoriatic arthritis

2. What investigation is likely to be diagnostic?

- ❑ A Joint aspirate and culture
- ❑ B MR scan
- ❑ C Clotting screen
- ❑ D Joint aspiration and polarised light microscopy
- ❑ E Complement levels

3. What therapy would you suggest?

- ❑ A Allopurinol
- ❑ B Diclofenac
- ❑ C Fresh frozen plasma
- ❑ D Co-amoxiclav
- ❑ E Methotrexate 60mg/week

Data Interpretation 5 (4 marks)

A 28-year-old woman with tuberose sclerosis presents with left-side pleuritic chest pain. Over the previous three months she has also developed an asymmetric polyarthropathy. On examination there is a fine pleural rub on the left and dullness to percussion at the right base. Mild synovitis is present in the joints of both hands. An auto-antibody screen reveals:

ANA	1:640
Anti-ds-DNA	1:1
Anti-histone	1:320
Anti-Sm	1:10
Rheumatoid factor	Negative
CRP	28 mg/l

1. What is the likely diagnosis?

❑ A Drug-induced lupus
❑ B Systemic lupus erythematodes
❑ C Paraneoplastic syndrome
❑ D Mixed connective tissue disease
❑ E Systemic sclerosis

2. What management would you recommend?

❑ A Aspirin
❑ B Chloroquine
❑ C Alter current medication
❑ D Oral steroids
❑ E Methotrexate

Data Interpretation 6 (4 marks)

A 26-year-old West Indian girl presents with a flitting arthritis affecting predominantly both ankles and her knees and hands. She has an intermittent low grade pyrexia and a dry cough. Investigations reveal:

Hb	124 g/l
WCC	12.1 x 10^9/l
Plt	437 x 10^9/l
ESR	88 mm/hr
Na	140 mmol/l
K	4.2 mmol/l
Urea	14.2 mmol/l
Calcium	2.6 mmol/l
Albumin	37 g/l
ANA	1:10
ASO	1:40
Rheumatoid factor	1:20

1. What is your next investigation?

- ❑ A Blood cultures
- ❑ B Chest X-ray
- ❑ C Throat swab
- ❑ D Radio-isotope bone scan
- ❑ E Serum ACE-levels

2. What is the likely diagnosis?

- ❑ A Systemic lupus erythematodes
- ❑ B Infective endocarditis
- ❑ C Non-Hodgkin lymphoma
- ❑ D Loefgren syndrome
- ❑ E Still's disease

Data Interpretation 7 (4 marks)

A 49-year-old woman presents with red eyes, a purpuric rash on both legs and polyarthralgia affecting the small joints of both hands.
A Schirmer test shows:

Left eye	2 mm/5 min (> 5 mm)
Right eye	3 mm/5 min (> 5 mm)

An auto-antibody screen shows:

Rheumatoid factor	> 1:5,000
Anti-nuclear antibodies	1:620
Anti-ds DNA	1:10
SS-A-(Ro) antibodies	1:320
SS-B-(La) antibodies	1:320

Hand X-ray: Normal bone density, no erosions

1. What is the likely diagnosis?

- ❑ A Rheumatoid arthritis
- ❑ B Mikulicz syndrome
- ❑ C Heerfordt syndrome
- ❑ D Systemic lupus erythematodes
- ❑ E Sjögren's syndrome

2. What therapy would you recommend?

- ❑ A Non-steroidal anti-inflammatory drugs
- ❑ B Oral steroids
- ❑ C Symptomatic therapy only
- ❑ D Plasmapheresis
- ❑ E Chloroquine

Data Interpretation 8 (5 marks)

A 17-year-old boy is being investigated for a swinging pyrexia and recurrent painful swelling of both knees. Over the last three weeks he has developed a sore red eye with acute visual deterioration over the preceding 24 hours. Blood samples reveal:

Hb	92g/l
MCV	78fl
WCC	19 x 10^9/l (94% neutrophils)
Plt	612 x 10^9/l
ESR	98mm/hr
Biochemical profile	Normal
Rheumatoid factor	1:10
Anti-nuclear antibodies (ANA)	1:160
Extractable nuclear antigen (ENA)	1:1
HLA B-27	Negative
Chest X-ray	Small right pleural effusion

1. **What is the likely diagnosis?**
2. **What is your immediate management?**

Data Interpretation 9 (4 marks)

A 56-year-old man is being assessed for a total knee replacement. The following results are obtained in the Orthopaedic Outpatient Department:

U&E's	Normal
Glucose	14.7 mmol/l
AST	51 U/l
ALT	72 U/l
Gamma GT	53 U/l
Bilirubin	16 µmol/l
Calcium	2.3 mmol/l
Ferritin	295 nmol/l (6–120 nmol/l)
Transferrin saturation	99%

Radiographs show advanced degenerative changes and chondrocalcinosis in both knees.

1. **What is the likely diagnosis?**

- ❑ A Acromegaly
- ❑ B Calcium pyrophosphate deposition disease
- ❑ C Chronic hepatic porphyria
- ❑ D Haemochromatosis
- ❑ E Neuropathic joint disease

2. **Which of the following investigations is likely to be diagnostic?**

- ❑ A Haemoglobin A1c
- ❑ B Liver biopsy
- ❑ C Joint aspirate
- ❑ D Oral glucose tolerance test
- ❑ E Faecal porphyrines

Data Interpretation 10 (6 marks)

A 73-year-old man presents with increasing shortness of breath, worse at night, and pain around the left hip joint. The following results are obtained:

FBC	Normal
ESR	16 mm/hr
U&E's	Normal
Calcium	2.35 mmol/l
Phosphate	1.2 mmol/l
Albumin	36 g/l
ALT	71 U/l
Gamma GT	89 U/l
Bilirubin	18 μmol/l
Alkaline phosphatase	1,190 U/l
Acid phosphatase	12 U/l (< 5 U/l)
Prostate specific antigen	1.9 ng/ml (< 1 ng/ml)
Urinary hydroxyproline	730 mmol/24 hr (70–300 mmol/24 hr)

1. What is the likely underlying diagnosis?

- ❑ A Paget's disease
- ❑ B Osteomalacia
- ❑ C Multiple myeloma
- ❑ D Liver cirrhosis
- ❑ E Carcinoma of prostate

2. What complication has occurred?

- ❑ A Stress fracture
- ❑ B Sarcomatous change
- ❑ C Hepatoma
- ❑ D Congestive cardiac failure
- ❑ E Metastatic disease

3. What investigation would you perform in the first instance?

- ❑ A Liver ultrasound and biopsy
- ❑ B Transrectal biopsy of prostate
- ❑ C Vitamin D levels
- ❑ D Serum and urine protein electrophoresis
- ❑ E Pelvic X-ray

Data Interpretation 11 (4 marks)

A 38-year-old woman presents with fatigue and increasing pain in both arms. On examination there is a mild bilateral polyarthritis affecting the arms and knees.

Blood pressure measurements:

Right arm	105/65 mmHg
Left arm	140/80 mmHg

Investigations show:

Hb	104 g/l
MCV	82 fl
WCC	12.4×10^9/l
Plt	481×10^9/l
ESR	68 mm/hr
Biochemical profile	Normal

1. What is the likely diagnostic?

❑ A Polymyalgia rheumatica
❑ B Coarctation
❑ C Polymyositis
❑ D Syphilitic aortitis
❑ E Takayasu's arteritis

2. What investigation is indicated?

❑ A Temporal artery biopsy
❑ B Muscle biopsy
❑ C Arch-aortogram
❑ D Contrast enhanced CT thorax
❑ E MR scan of aorta

Data Interpretation 12 (4 marks)

A 28-year-old woman is admitted with acute onset of shortness of breath, lower chest and epigastric pain. She is noticed to have peau d'orange on her neck. BP 95/65 mmHg, PR 100/min, no murmurs. The pedal pulses are absent.

ECG shows sinus tachycardia with left bundle branch block.

FBC	Normal
ESR	28 mm/hr
Na	136 mmol/l
K	4.1 mmol/l
Urea	8.5 mmol/l
Creatinine	123 µmol/l
Creatinine kinase	210 U/l
LDH	290 U/l
AST	38 U/l
Amylase	128 U/l

1. What is the underlying condition?

- ❑ A Kawasaki's disease
- ❑ B Pseudoxanthoma elasticum
- ❑ C Buerger's disease
- ❑ D Ehler-Danlos syndrome
- ❑ E Systemic sclerosis

2. What is the cause for her symptoms?

- ❑ A Aortic dissection
- ❑ B Bacterial endocarditis
- ❑ C Acute myocardial infarction
- ❑ D Rhabdomyolysis
- ❑ E Oesophageal dismotility

Data Interpretation 13 (4 marks)

A 56-year-old vagrant presents to Casualty complaining of pain in his right hip and difficulties getting up from a lying and squatting position. On examination he is cachectic with palmar erythema.

Investigations show:

Hb	106 g/l
WCC	3.2×10^9/l
Plt	142×10^9/l
MCV	102 fl
ESR	73 mm/hr
Na	132 mmol/l
K	3.1 mmol/l
Urea	2.8 mmol/l
Creatinine	153 µmol/l
Calcium	1.9 mmol/l
Phosphate	0.7 mmol/l
Albumin	28 g/l
ALT	116 U/l
Gamma GT	186 U/l
Bilirubin	21 µmol/l
Alkaline phosphate	563 U/l

1. What is the likely cause of the presenting symptoms?

- ❑ A Pathological fracture
- ❑ B Paraneoplastic syndrome
- ❑ C Myositis ossificans
- ❑ D Subacute combined degeneration of the cord
- ❑ E Osteomalacia

2. What is your next investigation?

- ❑ A C-reactive protein
- ❑ B Blood cultures
- ❑ C Lumbar puncture
- ❑ D Echocardiogram
- ❑ E Chest X-ray

Data Interpretation 14 (3 marks)

A 33-year-old Indian salesman presents with a 10-day history of low-grade pyrexia and polyarthralgia. On examination the left knee is hot with an effusion, and a pustular rash surrounding the joint. He has previously been well, except for an episode of non-specific urethritis 18-months previously.

Investigations show:

Biochemical profile	Normal
Glucose	6.4 mmol/l
CRP	43 mg/l
Auto-antibody screen	Negative
Rheumatoid factor	Negative
Joint aspirate	15 ml turbid fluid
Protein	53 g/l
Glucose	2.8 mmol/l
Culture	Negative

1. What is the likely diagnosis?

❑ A Pustular psoriasis
❑ B Reiter's syndrome
❑ C Secondary syphilis
❑ D Gonococcal arthritis
❑ E Tuberculous arthritis

2. What is your next investigation?

❑ A Blood cultures
❑ B Joint aspirate and culture
❑ C VDRL-test
❑ D Chest X-ray
❑ E Midstream urine sample

CARDIOLOGY ANSWERS: CASE HISTORIES

Answers – Case History 1 (9 marks)

1. A Mitral stenosis
2. E Mesenteric infarction
3. D Lactic acidosis
4. B Mesenteric angiogram

The patient has numerous features of **mitral stenosis**. Acute presentation with abdominal pain may indicate a posterior MI, however the patient also has a high anion gap acidosis ($[Na^+ + K^+] - [Cl^- + HCO_3^-] =$ 32 mmol/l). **Mesenteric infarction** causes a rise in lactate. A surgical opinion needs to be sought urgently. Plain abdominal films may be normal, an ultrasound scan may show a large loop of atonic bowel and some free fluid. However, the investigation of choice is angiography.

Answers – Case History 2 (8 marks)

1. C Coarctation
2. C Cardiac szintigraphy
3. B Noonan's syndrome
4. E Surgery

The patient has **coarctation**, which is one of the main differential diagnoses of hypertension and cardiac failure in a young patient. The post-ductal form is the more benign form presenting in adults, associated defects are PDA, VSD and bicuspid aortic valve (50%!). Pre- and post-stenotic dilatation of the aorta results in the 'figure of three' appearance of the chest X-ray. Collateral formation of intercostal vessels feeding the lower abdominal aorta results in inferior rib notching. Coarctation is commoner in males, and is associated with Turner's and Noonan's syndrome. Antibiotic prophylaxis is required until surgical correction has been performed.

Patients with Klinefelter's and homocysteinuria are of tall stature, Hurler's syndrome is a muco-polysaccharidosis with a poor prognosis, death occurs between 10 and 15 years of age.

Answers - Case History 3 (6 marks)

1. D Pericardial effusion
2. B Gout
3. E Thyroxine

The patient has clinical, cardiac, haematological and biochemical manifestations of **hypothyroidism**. Pericardial effusions in myxoedema respond well to thyroxine replacement and should not be drained. Post-viral pericardial effusion has to be considered, tuberculous and lymphomatous effusions are unlikely. Uraemia may cause pericardial effusion in end stages, gout does not.

Answers – Case History 4 (7 marks)

1. B DC-shocks, intubation and cardiac compressions
2. C Romano-Ward syndrome
3. D Torsade-de-Pointes tachycardia

Romano-Ward syndrome is one of the two congenital syndromes of prolonged QT-interval, which is autosomal d**o**minant with n**o**rmal hearing (J**e**rv**e**ll-Lang-Nielsen has r**e**c**e**ssive inheritance and neural d**e**afness). Torsade-de-Pointes arrhythmias are usually repetitive and self-terminating, but they can establish into VF. The QRS axis varies through the paroxysm. Acquired causes of QT prolongation include hypo-kalaemia, hypomagnesaemia, antihistamines, tricyclic antidepressants and some anti-arrhythmics (amiodarone, sotalol, flecainide).

TDP is resistant to DC-shocks and best treated with iv magnesium (1 ampoule, 8 mmol).

WPW and LGL are syndromes of accessory pathways. WPW is characterised by slurred R-upstrokes (delta waves). In Type **A** the QRS complex is **a**bove the baseline in V_1 (RBB pattern), in Type **B** the QRS complex is **b**elow the baseline (LBB pattern).

Answers – Case History 5 (8 marks)

1.
Best answer: **Perforation of ventricular septum**
Accepted answer: Ventricular septum defect
Rejected answer: Ruptured chordae tendineae/Mitral regurgitation

2.
Best answer: **Trans-thoracic echocardiogram**
Accepted answers: Echocardiogram/Left-sided cardiac catheter
Rejected answer: Trans-oesophageal echocardiogram/VQ scan

3.
Best answer: **Surgical repair/Cardiac surgery**
Rejected answer: Anticoagulation/Thrombolysis/Antibiotic prophylaxis

The presence of a significant **post-infarction VSD** is indicated by a high arterial pulmonary pressure, but normal wedge pressure and a high O_2-saturation indicating a left-to-right shunt. Other complications of MI include rupture of capillary muscle, ventricular rupture, LV aneurysm and post-infarction pericarditis (Dressler syndrome).

Answers – Case History 6 (6 marks)

1. D Renal artery stenosis
2. B Takayasu's arteritis

Takayasu's arteritis is a large vessel vasculitis resulting in narrowing and occlusion of large aortic branches and the pulmonary artery ('pulseless disease'). It typically affects young women and is commoner in Asian communities. Treatment with steroids shows success in most cases.

Kawasaki syndrome is a vasculitis which typically affects the coronary arteries, resulting in aneurysm formation. It occurs in children with a severe, systemic flu-like illness.

Pseudoxanthoma elasticum is associated with hypertension, aneurysm formation and ischaemic heart disease.

Answers – Case History 7 (10 marks)

1. D Echocardiogram, blood cultures and CT brain
2. B iv antibiotics and iv frusemide
3. A Endocarditis
4. B Cerebral abscess

Prophylaxis for **bacterial endocarditis** is currently recommended for high-risk patients (prosthetic valve, previous endocarditis) and the growing instrumentation of the GI, GU and respiratory tract as well as dental procedures. (Prophylaxis for barium enema is no longer recommended.) iv amoxicillin and iv gentamycin pre-procedure and oral amoxicillin post-procedure are currently regarded as adequate. Prophylaxis with oral amoxicillin only is adequate for patients with uncomplicated valvular lesions, septal defects and PDA undergoing simple dental procedures. Septic emboli to the brain are a serious complication that can lead to abscess formation.

Answers – Case History 8 (10 marks)

1. B Aortic dissection
2. A Myocardial infarction
   C Aortic incompetence
   G Left common carotid occlusion
3. A Blood cultures
4. E Marfan's syndrome

Dissection of the aorta may ascend from the root to involve the great vessels as well as the coronary arteries. The dilatation of the ascending aorta causes aortic incompetence by dilatation of the valve rings.

The patient has an inferior infarction, the raised JVP may be due to compromise of the right ventricle or haemorrhage into the mediastinum. Normal heart sounds and jugular venous wave form are against pericardial haemorrhage. The cardiac complications account for the reduced life expectancy in **Marfan's syndrome**, the patients often die in their forties. Other features include upper dislocation of the lens of the eye, angioid streaks, increased arm span and arachnodactyly, high arched palate and recurrent pneumothoraces.

Answers – Case History 9 (5 marks)

1. D Auto-immune pericarditis
2. C Indomethacin

Post-cardiotomy syndrome occurs up to one year following cardiac surgery. It is an acute febrile illness with pericarditis and/or pleuritis. Pleural and pericardial effusions are frequently found. The disease, similar to Dressler's syndrome (pericarditis two to four weeks after MI), is usually self-limiting but may require treatment with non-steroidal anti-inflammatories or, if these fail, steroids. Pericarditic pain is typically worse lying down and relieved by sitting forward. Typical ECG changes of pericarditis may be subtle or absent in the auto-immune form.

Answers – Case History 10 (7 marks)

1. C Echocardiogram
2. E Ebstein's anomaly
3. B AV re-entrant tachycardia

Ebstein's anomaly is characterised by a low insertion of the tricuspid valve resulting in a large atrium and a small, hypoplastic ventricle ('atrialisation' of right ventricle). This spectrum of the disease is broad, ranging from incidental findings at post-mortem to early, severe presentations in childhood. Common associated findings are tricuspid incompetence, atrial septal defect (leading to cyanosis) and accessory conduction pathways. WPW syndrome is found in up to 10%. Supraventricular tachycardias are common, usually due to retrograde conduction through the accessory bundle leading to re-entrant tachycardia. Diagnosis is by transthoracic echocardiogram.

Answers – Case History 11 (7 marks)

1.
Best answers: **Cortical blindness/Occipital infarction/Vertebro-basilar embolus**
Accepted answer: Cerebral embolus
Rejected answer: Amaurosis fugax/Retinal embolus

2.
Best answer: **Left atrial myxoma**
Accepted answers: Atrial myxoma/Atrial thrombus
Rejected answers: Mitral stenosis

Atrial myxoma is a benign, gelatinous tumour arising from the septum. It is three times more common on the left-side and is frequently associated with a raised ESR, raised globulins and may have associated systemic symptoms. Embolisation is common, treatment is by surgical resection. Echocardiogram shows a high echogenicity tumour in the atrium. During diastole it partially prolapses through the valve, resulting in a third heart sound, 'tumour plop'.

Infarction of the occipital cortex results in disturbed processing of the visual input, the patient may not be aware of the visual deficit.

Answers - Case History 12 (8 marks)

1. B Nephroblastoma (Wilms' tumour)
2. B Urinary catecholamines
3. E iv rehydration and α-blockade

Only approximately 50% of patients with **phaeochromocytoma** present with episodic hypertension, 50% of adults and up to 90% of children present with sustained hypertension which may remain unnoticed for a long period of time. Drug abuse may result in hypertensive crises, but is unlikely to result in left ventricular hypertrophy. 10% of phaeo's are malignant/bilateral/familial/extra-adrenal. Thoracic phaeo's tend to secrete nor-adrenaline only. The patients require α-blockade prior to surgery to prevent a hypertensive crisis and aggressive rehydration to prevent post-operative hypotension. Fibro-muscular renal artery stenosis may present in younger patients, as may Conn's syndrome, the key feature being hypokalaemia. Nephroblastoma is a malignant embryological tumour of the kidney which usually presents before the age of five with a large renal mass and haematuria.

CARDIOLOGY ANSWERS: DATA INTERPRETATIONS

Answers – Data Interpretation 1 (4 marks)

1. B Significant ischaemia
2. E Coronary angiography

There is a ST-segment depression of >1 mm in leads II, III, aVF and V_{3-6} at 0.8 second after the 'J' point. This is a strongly **positive exercise test** and suggests multi-vessel disease because of involvement of anterior and inferior leads. This requires further investigation and treatment.

Answer – Data Interpretation 2 (3 marks)

1. C Prinzmetal (variant) angina

There is intermittent ST segment elevation (at 09.33 and 09.53) as well as ST depression 10.13). **Variant angina** is due to coronary spasm, often also associated with atheromatous disease. It typically occurs at night or in the early hours and is more common in women.

Answer – Data Interpretation 3 (2 marks)

1. D Fallot's tetralogy

The pressure in the right ventricle is higher than in the left ventricle, however pulmonary artery pressure is normal. There must be pulmonary stenosis. A right to left shunt is required to cause cyanosis, the most likely explanation is **Fallot's tetralogy** (pulmonary stenosis, right ventricular hypertrophy, ventricular septum defect with the aortic root overriding the VSD).

Answers – Data Interpretation 4 (5 marks)

1. E Coarctation and bicuspid aortic valve
2. B Chromosomal analysis

The patient has **Turner's syndrome**. Over one-third of patients have coarctation, this is associated with a bicuspid aortic valve. Diagnosis can simply be made on a buccal smear which shows the absence of a Barr body. A hand X-ray may show short 4th and 5th metacarpals, this is also a feature of pseudohypoparathyroidism and pseudo-pseudohypoparathyroidism.

Answers – Data Interpretation 5 (4 marks)

1. C Right ventricular infarction
2. A Thrombosis of right coronary artery

The right ventricular filling pressure is high, while left ventricular filling pressure (pulmonary capillary wedge pressure) is low. This indicates that predominantly the right ventricle is affected. The sinus node is supplied by a branch of the right coronary artery.

Answers – Data Interpretation 6 (5 marks)

1.
Best answers: **Grand-mal seizure/Epileptic fit**
Accepted answer: Rhabdomyolysis
Rejected answer: Myocardial infarction

2.
Best answers: **Creatinine kinase iso-enzymes/Troponine T levels**
Accepted answer: Serial ECGs
Rejected answer: Serial cardiac enzymes

Cardiac muscle has a higher AST content than **skeletal muscle** and in myocardial infarction the levels of AST are usually at least 10% of that of the CK. An extremely high CK with a relatively low AST indicates skeletal muscle damage. The estimation of creatinine kinase is being superseded by troponine T, which is more specific and has a higher predictive value for outcome. However, it is currently more expensive and not yet widely available. It may have false negative values in the first 12 hours.

Answers – Data Interpretation 7 (5 marks)

1. E Patent ductus arteriosus
2. D Angiographic embolization

PDA may be an isolated defect, and if small, may be discovered as an incidental finding. Large PDAs without pressure reduction result in secondary pulmonary hypertension and shunt reversal, if untreated. Compensating PDAs (i.e. with associated pulmonary stenosis/atresia) may represent a life-saving left-to-right shunt and closure may be prevented by prostaglandin E1. Prostacyclin inhibitors (NSAID) may be used as a conservative attempt for closure of a PDA, particularly in premature babies. All PDAs require endocarditis prophylaxis.

Answers – Data Interpretation 8 (5 marks)

1. A Dilating (congestive) cardiomyopathy
2. E Alcohol abuse

The patient has cardiomegaly with a poor ejection fraction ('a large floppy heart'). HOCM and aortic stenosis show concentric hypertrophy of the myocardium with only dilatation in the final stages. Restrictive cardiomyopathy is a rare condition with endocardial fibrosis, the main differential being constrictive pericarditis.

Causes of **dilating cardiomyopathy** include auto-immune, post-viral, drug-induced (cytotoxic and tricyclic antidepressants) and alcohol. The patient has macrocytic anaemia which tips the balance towards a social cause.

Answers – Data Interpretation 9 (4 marks)

1. C 2° heart block
2. A Observation only

The patient has a **2°AV-block** heart block with **Wenckebach periodicity** (Mobitz 1). The PR interval increases until one QRS complex is dropped. This has a better prognosis than a Mobitz 2 block with a fixed conduction deficit. Asymptomatic patients do not require treatment.

Answer – Data Interpretation 10 (3 marks)

1.

Best answer: **Acute postero-inferior infarction**
Accepted answers: Acute inferior infarction/Acute posterior infarction
Rejected answer: Pericarditis

ST elevation in inferior leads is obvious, however there is ST depression in the anterior chest leads giving the mirror image of a posterior wall infarction.

Answers – Data Interpretation 11 (5 marks)

1. C Wolff-Parkinson-White Type A
2. E Left-sided accessory bundle

There is a short PR interval and a slurred upstroke of the R-wave (Δ-wave). In addition there is RBB pattern in V_1 and V_2 with an M-shaped, positive deflection indicating **WPW type A**. (Type A = QRS above baseline). This occurs because the left-sided Kent bundle excites the left ventricle before the right, the appearance being of a relative conduction delay to the right ventricle (RBB). Conversely, in Type B there is normal appearance in V_1 (Type B = QRS below baseline) with a LBB pattern, because the right-sided Kent bundle triggers the right ventricle prior to the left.

Answers – Data Interpretation 12 (4 marks)

1. D Mitral stenosis
2. C Pulmonary hypertension

There is increased pressure in the left atrium, the lungs and the right heart. The gradient between the atrial pressure and the diastolic pressure in the left ventricle indicates **mitral stenosis**. There is also a significant pressure gradient across the pulmonary capillary bed. The pulmonary vascular resistance (PVR) can be calculated as the mean pressure difference between pulmonary artery and left atrium, divided by the cardiac output. In this case it is 24/3 = 8. Normal PVR is < 1, values > 8 indicate high risk for surgery.

Answers – Data Interpretation 13 (6 marks)

1.

Best answer: **(Coarse) ventricular fibrillation**
Accepted answers: Ventricular tachycardia/Torsades-de-Pointes tachycardia
Rejected answers: Atrial flutter/Supra-ventricular tachycardia

2.

Best answer: **DC-shocks (200J, 200J, 360J)**
Accepted answer: Synchronised cardio-version
Rejected answers: Precordial thump/iv magnesium

3.
Best answer: **Acute posterior myocardial infarction**
Accepted answer: Posterior myocardial infarction
Rejected answer: Septal ischaemia/Left bundle branch block

Management of cardiac arrest is an infrequent, but recurring theme of the exam. Detailed knowledge of the latest guidelines will be expected by the examiners, in particular in the clinical part of the exam.

Answer – Data Interpretation 14 (3 marks)

1. D Aortic stenosis

The ECG shows a mild bradycardia, a normal QRS axis, but marked left ventricular hypertrophy. The Sokolow-index (S_{V2} + R_{V5}) is over 70 mm. There is descending ST depression in the lateral leads in keeping with left ventricular strain, however the deep T-inversion is also suspicious for a recent sub-endocardial infarct.

Aortic stenosis can go undetected for a remarkably long period of time, as the heart is much better at compensating for a pressure load than a volume load. Cardiomegaly in the chest X-ray ensues with decompensation. HOCM would also have to be considered, although they tend to present earlier and have a strong family history (autosomal dominant).

Answer – Data Interpretation 15 (2 marks)

1. C Carotid dissection

Electro-mechanical dissociation ('normal' ECG without output) can be caused by the following mechanisms – massive haemorrhage and hypovolaemia, cardiac outflow obstruction (massive PE, air embolism, failing prosthetic valve), cardiac tamponade, tension pneumothorax, hypothermia and drug overdose. Carotid dissection can occur after trivial trauma to the neck and is one of the leading causes for stroke in young patients.

Answers – Data Interpretation 16 (5 marks)

1. E Complete heart block
2. A Thrombolysis

The patient has two (pain, enzyme rise) out of three criteria for **acute infarction** as well as an abnormal ECG. Complete heart block indicates an inferior infarct. Prognosis of this is usually good with recovery within two weeks. Unless the patient is haemodynamically compromised, pacing should be withheld.

Answers – Data Interpretation 17 (5 marks)

1. D Ostium secundum atrial septal defect
2. A Ventilation perfusion lung scan

There is a step-up of saturation in the right atrium, indicating a left-to-right shunt. However, of the four options given for a defect at this level, the ECG changes indicate an **ASD**. By far the commoner form is an ostium secundum defect which is also likely to present later on in life. Paradoxical emboli to the systemic circulation can be found despite the predominant left-to-right shunt. Injection of embolising particles (microalbumin aggregates) in a lung perfusion scan is therefore contra-indicated, they usually end up in the brain or in the kidneys.

Answers – Data Interpretation 18 (4 marks)

1 A Left anterior descending artery
2. D Aspirin and r-TPA

The patient has an acute **anterior myocardial infarction**. In a young patient, the thrombolytic agent of choice is r-TPA.

Answer – Data Interpretation 19 (3 marks)

1.
Best answer: **Limb-lead reversal**
Accepted answer: Lead reversal ECG
Rejected answers: Anterior MI/Pulmonary embolus/Dextrocardia

There is complete inversion of the trace in lead I and AVL with normal appearances in the chest leads. The P-axis is in the region of 110–120° without evidence of abnormal atrial conduction.

Answers – Data Interpretation 20 (4 marks)

1. B Renal tubular acidosis Type I
2. A Abdominal X-ray

The patient has ECG evidence of hypokalaemia. This is unusual to be combined with a metabolic acidosis. Flank pain and haematuria indicate renal stones. The diagnosis is **distal renal tubular acidosis (Type 1)**. The most sensitive way of detecting stones is a simple X-ray. Confirmation is with an acid-load challenge, the ammonium chloride test. The kidneys will fail to acidify the urine below a pH of 5.4.

Answers – Data Interpretation 21 (5 marks)

1. C Toxic cardiomyopathy
2. B Venesection

The patient has **haemochromatosis**. The cardinal features are diabetes, liver disease and skin pigmentation (beware the well-looking patient!). Myocardial deposition of iron leads to a dilating cardiomyopathy. Initial therapy is with iron removal by blood letting.

Answers – Data Interpretation 22 (4 marks)

1. E Mobitz Type 2 heart block
2. C Sarcoidosis

The ECG shows a **2° AV-Block** with variable transmission (Mobitz 2). This indicates organic heart disease. Cardiac involvement is rare in **sarcoidosis** (< 5%). Conduction defects, arrhythmias and cardiomyopathy are seen. Polydipsia and polyuria are signs of the associated hypercalcaemia.

Answers – Data Interpretation 23 (5 marks)

1. D Hypertrophic obstructive cardiomyopathy
2. B Friedreich's ataxia

The relentlessly progressive **Friedreich's ataxia** manifests in childhood or adolescence with progressive ataxia. Inheritance is autosomal recessive. Pes cavus, the mixture of lower and upper motor neurone signs and marked cerebellar signs are typical. Cardiac involvement results in cardiomyopathy, HOCM, arrhythmias and left ventricular hypertrophy.

Answer – Data Interpretation 24 (3 marks)

1.

Best answer: **Ventricular septal defect with shunt reversal/ Eisenmenger complex**

Accepted answers: Ventricular septum defect/Eisenmenger syndrome

Rejected answer: Atrial septal defect

Congenital cardiac defects are common in chromosomal anomalies. The patient has a step-down of saturation in the left ventricle with a slight increase in left-sided pressures. Eponyms should be generally avoided, but Eisenmenger *complex* indicates shunt reversal associated with VSD. Eisenmenger *syndrome* denotes the reversal of a left-to-right shunt due to the development of pulmonary hypertension without specifying the underlying cause. At this stage, the patients are inoperable.

ENDOCRINOLOGY ANSWERS: CASE HISTORIES

Answers – Case History 1 (9 marks)

1. B Secondary hyperthyroidism
2. C MR scan of pituitary
3. D Carbimazole
4. C Transsphenoidal hypophysectomy

A raised TSH in the presence of a raised T4 indicates failure of the feedback to the pituitary and the presence of either a **secondary (pituitary) hyperthyroidism** or ectopic TSH production (trophoblastic disease). The latter is unlikely as the patient is on oral contraceptives. In primary (thyroid) hyperthyroidism, TSH and TRH would be suppressed, in tertiary (hypothalamic) hyperthyroidism, the TRH would be high, stimulating TSH and T4 secretion.

Increased secretion of TSH by the pituitary is usually due to an adenoma but may occur as 'simple' hypersecretion.

Pituitary adenomata, if very small, may even be missed by MRI scanning, however the differentiation from TSH hypersecretion of the gland may be demonstrated by failure of TSH to suppress with bromocriptine and failure to increase in the TRH test. Conservative treatment (bromocriptine, octreotide) may be successful, but surgery will often be required.

Treatment of the end-organ thyroid with carbimazole, surgery or radio-iodine will only show transient response as the maintained stimulation with TSH will facilitate re-growth of any residual thyroid tissue.
Patients on thyrostatics need to be monitored for agranulocytosis.

Answers – Case History 2 (10 marks)

1. C Primary hyperparathyroidism
2. D Technetium-MIBI-subtraction scan

Three causes account for 70% of bilateral medullary nephrocalcinosis:

- Primary hyperparathyroidism
- Medullary sponge kidney
- Renal tubular acidosis Type I

The patient, besides being hypercalcaemic, also has recurrent duodenal ulcers and evidence of bone resorption indicating hyperparathyroidism. Assessment of hyperparathyroidism in the first instance is with Technetium-MIBI-subtraction scan and ultrasound of the neck. (Cesta-MIBI is taken up by parathyroid as well as thyroid gland, from this scan a pure thyroid Technetium scan is subtracted. Areas of increased activity on the subtraction scan indicate hyperactive parathyroid tissue.)

3. A MR pituitary and CT pancreas
4. C Wermer syndrome (multiple endocrine neoplasia Type I)
5. D Glucagonoma

Bi-temporal hemianopia indicates compression of the optic chiasm, direct imaging of this area is required.

Unusual rashes are seen with pancreatic tumours. Erythema gyratum repens and wandering thrombophlebitis are paraneoplastic manifestations of carcinoma of the pancreas. However, a migrating necrotizing rash is seen typically with glucagonoma.

Patients with **MEN Type I** (autosomal dominant) develop a variety of pancreatic tumours, in particular glucagonoma, vipoma, insulinoma and gastrinoma. The pancreas is best assessed with thin sections of a dynamic contrast-enhanced CT. (P. Wermer, US physician)

The hyperparathyroidism in MEN Type I is more often due to parathyroid hyperplasia; in Type II more often due to parathyroid adenoma, but variation is considerable.

MEN Type IIa consists of phaeochromocytoma, hyperparathyroidism and medullary carcinoma of the thyroid. This may be associated with hamarfanoid habitus and skin neurinomata reminiscent of neurofibromatosis and is then termed MEN Type IIb.

Answers – Case History 3 (9 marks)

1. A Impaired glucose tolerance

There is a slow rise in the glucose which does not reach diabetic levels, but remains higher than 8 mmol/l at two hours.

2. C Adrenal adenoma and ectopic ACTH secretion

The base line cortisol is raised. It does not suppress in the extended (high dose) dexamethasone test. These are the features of either a **primary adrenal tumour** or **ectopic ACTH secretion**. Pituitary driven (Cushing's disease) and hyperthalamic driven hypercortisolism both suppress in the high dose dexamethasone test. Factitious cortisol administration cannot be excluded on the basis of this test, however the history indicates that this is a long-standing process and no suitable combination of answers is available.

3. E Serum ACTH levels

Adrenal adenoma and ectopic ACTH secretion are easily distinguished by estimating the serum ACTH which would be extremely low in case of an adrenal adenoma or carcinoma, as the pituitary would be suppressed by the high levels of cortisol.

Ectopic ACTH secretion and pituitary driven hyperadrenalism can also be distinguished by the CRH test which leads to a further increase in plasma ACTH in the central form, with ectopic ACTH secretion the pituitary is completely suppressed and will not respond to CRH.

Long-term therapy with systemic steroids will, of course, also suppress endogenous ACTH and cortisol production.

4. C Acute adrenal failure

The patient is in Addisonian crisis, as the endogenous ACTH/cortisol production will have been chronically suppressed by either an adenoma or ectopic ACTH secretion.

Answers – Case History 4 (8 marks)

1. C Radio-isotope bone scan
2. D Metastatic carcinoma
3. A Leukoerythroblastic film due to bone marrow invasion
4. A iv saline

The patient presents with symptoms of hypercalcaemia. The following causes usually suppress to normal levels with oral steroids: sarcoidosis, myeloma, hypervitaminosis, and Addison's disease. Ectopic PTH production and bone metastases suppress to variable degree, hyperparathyroidism is not affected.

Hyperparathyroidism is also ruled out by the high phosphate. The low globulin fraction (total protein – albumin) and low ESR are against myeloma.

The patient has erythroid and myeloid precursors in the bloodstream indicating bone marrow invasion (or myelofibrosis).

In combination, this makes a **metastasised carcinoma** with bone metastases (the patient has back pain) and bone marrow invasion the most likely cause. In a female of that age, the likely primaries are breast and bronchus.

Treatment of hypercalcaemia is with hyperhydration with intravenous saline – cardiac and renal function allowing. Addition of loop diuretics (furosemide) will increase renal excretion of calcium.

Treatment with diphosphonates is a further option, steroids can be used in hypercalcaemia due to myeloma.

Answers – Case History 5 (10 marks)

1. B 240

The serum osmolality is calculated as follows (Na + K) x 2 + urea + glucose.

2. E Inappropriate ADH secretion

The patient has extremely low osmolality of the serum with an inappropriately high osmolality of the urine. Causes for **inappropriate ADH secretion** include any intracranial pathology (tumour, hydrocephalus, infection), intrathoracic pathology (tumour, empyema, infection, in particular Legionella), a number of drugs (in particular, drugs beginning with 'c', i.e. chlorpropamide, chlorothiazide, cytotoxics and carbamazepine) as well as lymphoma and acute intermittent porphyria.

3. D Fluid restriction and iv diazepam

The treatment for SIADH is fluid restriction. The patient, however, is in status epilepticus and requires appropriate treatment.

4. B Central pontine myelinolysis

5. B MR brain

Rapid correction of the electrolyte disturbance is contra-indicated. The change in blood results suggests that the patient has been given (hypertonic) saline intravenously with a disastrous result. The posterior fossa and the brain stem are poorly demonstrated on CT but will be clearly shown on MR scanning.

Answers – Case History 6 (8 marks)

1. B Primary hypothyroidism
2. E MR scan of pituitary
3. A Increased TRH production
4. C Oral thyroxine

The patient has multiple clinical stigmata of **hypothyroidism**, including a macrocytic anaemia and evidence of a pericardial effusion. This is supported by the biochemistry which indicates primary thyroid failure with a raised TSH as the pituitary is trying to stimulate thyroxine production. The presence of thyroid antibodies confirms the autoimmune aetiology.

Long-standing, untreated hypothyroidism will lead to hyperplasia of the pituitary, which can lead to compression of the optic chiasm and, rarely, to secondary pituitary failure. However, there is no other evidence of end-organ failure, gonadotrophins and cortisol are normal. Increased release of thyrotrophin from the hypothalamus also stimulates release of prolactin from the anterior pituitary. Thyroid replacement therapy will remove the stimulus to the pituitary, which will reduce in size, and prolactin levels will drop.

Answers – Case History 7 (13 marks)

1.
Best answer: **Congenital adrenal hyperplasia**
Accepted answer: Increased testosterone
Rejected answers: Conn's syndrome/Polycystic ovary syndrome

2.
Best answers: **Mineralocorticoid effect (of 11-deoxycorticosterone)/ Excess aldosterone precursors**
Accepted answer: Hyper-aldosteronism
Rejected answers: Adrenal adenoma/Renal artery stenosis

3.
Best answer: **Likelihood not increased**
Rejected answer: Increased likelihood

4.
Best answers: **Adrenal substitution/Mineralo-plus glucocorticoid administration**
Rejected answers: Adenectomy/Adrenalectomy/Hypophysectomy

Hypertension in the presence of hypokalaemia in a young patient should always alert to the possibility of Conn's syndrome. However, the fact that the patient has evidence of virilization and the unusual endocrine tests suggests an alternative diagnosis.

The patient has excess testosterone with suppression of the gonadotrophins. In addition, there is evidence of hyper-aldosteronism with high Na, low K and a suppressed renin.

Congenital adrenal hyperplasia, CAH (also adreno-genital syndrome, AGS) is an inherited enzyme defect in the production of corticosteroids in the adrenal gland. The two main sites at the level of the 21-beta-hydroxylase (90%) and one step further down in the synthesis at 11-beta-hydroxylase (5%). In the commoner form, no functional precursors are produced and, as well as features of hypocortisonalism, the patients have evidence of salt wastage. In the second form, a functioning mineralocorticoid precursor (11-deoxycorticosterone) is produced leading to functional hyper-aldosteronism.

The absence of glucocorticoids leads to a reactive increase of ACTH secretion which stimulates the attempted production of the hormones. As all the corticoid precursors accumulate, there is further increase in androgen synthesis. This results in pseudopubertas praecox in boys and virilization in girls. The patients are initially tall but, due to premature fusion of the physes, end up with a reduced body height. Treatment is with substitution of the missing hormones, with the aim to suppress ACTH production to remove the stimulus to the adrenal. Family screening is also required as some forms can remain subclinical.

Answers – Case History 8 (7 marks)

1.
Best answer: **Hereditary vitamin D dependent rickets**
Accepted answer: Vitamin D dependent rickets
Rejected answers: Familial hypophosphataemic rickets/ Hyperparathyroidism/Pseudo-hypoparathyroidism

2.
Best answer: **Response to exogenous vitamin D**
Accepted answer: Vitamin D levels
Rejected answers: Examination of small bowel/Liver biopsy/Renal biopsy

The results are of a hypocalcaemia with secondary hyperparathyroidism (in primary hyperparathyroidism, there would be elevation of the calcium). The radiograph is typical for rickets. The family history suggests a congenital, possibly a familial disorder (confirmed by the third question). The history also leads away from common causes of vitamin D deficiency, such as poor diet, malabsorption and drug-induced.

The differential now lies between vitamin D dependent rickets (autosomal recessive) and familial hypophosphataemic rickets (X-linked dominant). Vitamin D **dependent** rickets has two types. The much more common Type I has a failure of 1-hydroxylation of cholecalciferol in the kidney. Serum levels of 1,25-$(OH)_2$-D are <u>low</u>. There is excellent response to small doses of exogenous vitamin D and 1α-OH-D. In the rarer Type II, there is end-organ resistance to 1,25-$(OH)_2$-D and serum levels are <u>high</u>. In familial hypophosphataemic rickets (vitamin D **resistant** rickets) there is profound renal tubular loss of phosphate with a relatively normal calcium. The parathormone is normal. Treatment here is with oral phosphate, as well as vitamin D. Due to the calcium/phosphate imbalance, there is secondary end-organ resistance to vitamin D.

3.
Best answer: **Autosomal recessive**
Accepted answer: Recessive inheritance
Rejected answers: Dominant inheritance/X-linked recessive inheritance

Assuming the data given are correct, the disease has been passed with male-to-male transmission from grandfather to grandson, skipping a generation. Skipping a generation indicates a recessive disorder, which suggests that both parents are carriers of the faulty gene.

ENDOCRINOLOGY ANSWERS: DATA INTERPRETATIONS

Answer – Data Interpretation 1 (2 marks)

1. C Pseudohypoparathyroidism Type I

Parathormone increases the urinary phosphate excretion. This is mediated within the cell by the second messenger c-AMP. After infusion of intravenous PTH, urinary excretion of c-AMP and phosphate should increase by the factor 10-15. In hypoparathyroidism, there is not enough endogenous parathormone. In **pseudohypoparathyroidism**, there is end-organ resistance within the kidney to PTH. In Type I, there is a complete receptor defect and neither c-AMP nor phosphate excretion is increased. In Type II, the cell receptor is intact and c-AMP rises, with the consequent increase in urinary excretion, but phosphate levels do not change.

Pseudohypoparathyroidism is associated with somatic features (short stature, moon face, short 4th and 5th metacarpal and intellectual impairment). In addition, ectopic soft tissue calcification is found more commonly in Type I than in Type II. In pseudo-pseudohypoparathyroidism, the skeletal abnormalities are found, but the biochemistry is normal.

Answer – Data Interpretation 2 (2 marks)

1. C Self-administration of insulin

The patient has a raised insulin in the presence of hypoglycaemia. C-peptide which is produced by cleavage of pro-insulin, however, is reduced indicating that the insulin present is exogenous insulin. In sulphonylurea overdose, pro-insulin, C-peptide and insulin are raised which can make differentiation from an insulinoma difficult.

Answers – Data Interpretation 3 (5 marks)

1. E Acromegaly
2. D Compression of pituitary stalk

The patient has *manifest* diabetes and shows a paradoxical rise of growth hormone in the oral glucose tolerance test, indicating **acromegaly**.
The excretion of prolactin is regulated by secretion of prolactin-inhibiting hormone (PIH = dopamine). Supra-sellar extension of a pituitary tumour may compress the pituitary infundibulum and PIH cannot reach the anterior pituitary which results in an uninhibited production of prolactin.

Answers – Data Interpretation 4 (4 marks)

1. B Klinefelter's syndrome
2. E Testosterone replacement

The presence of Barr bodies in a man indicates an extra X-chromosome in keeping with **Klinefelter's syndrome** (47 XXY). This is confirmed by an increased lower/upper body segment ratio (normal less than one). The patient would also have gynaecomastia and underdeveloped external genitalia. Klinefelter patients are infertile. There is a deficiency of androgens leading to an increased growth of long bones. The result is a eunuchoid growth pattern with increased arm span and long legs. Testicular biopsy shows fibrosis and hyalinisation of the seminiferous tubules which results in small, firm testes and azoospermia, but this is not diagnostic of the condition. Some patients may show a mosaic pattern in the chromosomal analysis/mixture of (46 XY and 47 XXY) leading to a milder expression of the disease with preserved fertility in some individuals. Treatment is with depot injections of testosterone which will produce virilization and prevent osteoporosis, but fertility cannot be restored.

Testicular feminization is an end-organ resistance to androgens leading to completed development of secondary female characteristics. The patients grow up normally as girls until investigations for amenorrhoea reveal the male genome (46 XY).

Answers – Data Interpretation 5 (4 marks)

1.
Best answer: **T3 thyrotoxicosis**
Accepted answer: Hyperthyroidism
Rejected answer: Pituitary failure

2.
Best answer: **Increased thyroxine-binding globulin**
Accepted answer: Spurious result
Rejected answer: Hyperthyroidism

T3 thyrotoxicosis is characterised by a normal free T4 concentration, but an elevated free T3 concentration (which is the investigation of choice). As in 'normal' hyperthyroidism, TSH levels are suppressed and fail to increase after administration of TRH.

In addition, this patient has an increase in hepatic synthesis of TBG due to the oestrogens contained in the contraceptive pill. T3 thyrotoxicosis is seen more frequently in patients with thyroid adenomas/multi-nodular goitres than in Graves' disease.

Answers – Data Interpretation 6 (4 marks)

1. D Peripheral diabetes insipidus
2. A No change

The patient has a plasma osmolality that rises with water deprivation rapidly above normal levels while the urine osmolality remains inappropriately low. The patient is losing water which indicates diabetes insipidus.

In the context given, the patient is *most likely* to have drug-induced (i.e. lithium) **peripheral diabetes insipidus** where there is resistance of the kidney to endogenous (and exogenous) anti-diuretic hormone. In this case, injection of synthetic ADH will also have no significant effect on the urine osmolality. Other causes for nephrogenic DI include chronic hypokalaemia and hypercalcaemia, other drugs, such as demeclocycline, amphotericin B and a rare X-linked recessive form which requires early treatment to prevent mental and physical impairment.

In central diabetes insipidus, there is failure of the posterior pituitary to produce ADH. The patients equally fail to retain water and, under water deprivation, the serum plasma osmolality rises above 300. However, after injection of DDAVP, there is an increase in the urine osmolality > 15%. DDAVP can be administered therapeutically as a nasal spray.
Psychogenic polydipsia is not a differential diagnosis as the patient starts with a high normal plasma osmolality (normal 270–295 mosmol/kg) and, by definition, has therefore not diluted himself.

Answer – Data Interpretation 7 (3 marks)

1. D Familial hypocalciuric hypercalcaemia

This is an autosomal dominant condition, characterised by increased renal absorption of calcium and magnesium. A mild hypermagnesaemia is seen in approximately 50%. The parathormone level is reduced, the other electrolytes are normal. Other causes of hypercalcaemia and renal tubular acidosis show an increased urinary calcium.

Answers – Data Interpretation 8 (5 marks)

1.

Best answers:	**Urinary catecholamines/Ultrasound scan neck/ Ultrasound or CT adrenals/Parathormone levels**
Accepted answers:	Calcitonin levels/Ultrasound kidneys/Family history
Rejected answers:	Sputum examination/Adrenaline levels/CT neck

2.

Best answer:	**Multiple endocrine neoplasia Type II**
Accepted answer:	Multiple endocrine neoplasia
Rejected answers:	Multiple endocrine neoplasia Type I/Malignant phaeochromocytoma

MEN Type II (Sipple syndrome) is the autosomal dominant syndrome of primary hyperparathyroidism (more commonly adenoma), phaeochromocytoma and medullary carcinoma of the thyroid (J.H. Sipple, US chest physician). If associated with marfanoid habitus and multiple neurinoma of skin and mucous membranes, it is termed 'Type II (b)'. Medullary carcinoma of the thyroid on its own is also transmitted as an autosomal dominant trait.

MEN Type I (Wermer syndrome), also autosomal dominant, is a combination of primary hyperparathyroidism (more commonly hyperplasia), variable pancreatic tumours (gastrinoma, glucagonoma, insulinoma, etc.) and pituitary tumours.

Answers – Data Interpretation 9 (6 marks)

1. A Subacute thyroiditis
2. C Fine needle aspirate and systemic steroids
3. D Hypothyroidism

The patient has evidence of active thyroiditis, however the white cells are not elevated indicating **subacute thyroiditis (de Quervain)**. This is characterised by raised ESR, raised T3 and T4 levels due to liberation of the hormones from the inflamed gland, which suppresses TSH. Prognosis is very good and most patients do not require treatment and, despite initial hyperthyroid status, return to normal function. However, hypothyroidism may ensue and, if severe, the patient may be treated with steroids.

Acute bacterial thyroiditis, of course, requires antibiotics and aspiration of any collections. Chronic lymphocytic thyroiditis (Hashimoto's) occurs in middle-aged women, is associated with thyroid auto-antibodies. There is insidious onset of hypothyroidism which, potentially, leads to firm fibrosis of the gland (Riedel's goitre). Fine needle aspirate is a safe procedure when done under ultrasound control.

Answers – Data Interpretation 10 (5 marks)

1.

Best answers:	**a. Prolactinoma**
	b. Panhypopituitarism
Accepted answer:	Pituitary failure
Rejected answer:	Hypothalamic dysfunction

2.

Best answers:	**Assess adrenal axis/Synacthen® test**
Accepted answers:	9 am cortisol/MR or CT scan of pituitary/Visual field examination
Rejected answer:	Lateral skull X-ray

GH fails to increase by 15 mU/l rise above 20 mU/l despite adequate hypoglycaemia (2.2 mmol/l or less). TSH is low and does not show a sustained elevation (30 min peak should be 5 mU/l or more above baseline, 60 min value at least 60% of 30 min value). LH is slow and shows poor response. Prolactin is in diagnostic range (> 5,000 U/l) for **prolactinoma** and shows only minimal increase after TRH. It is vital to assess the adrenal axis, as steroids will have to be replaced before thyroxine in order to prevent an acute Addisonian crisis.

Answers – Data Interpretation 11 (5 marks)

1. D Cushing's syndrome
2. E Long-term steroid therapy

In the short Synacthen® test, plasma cortisol should rise by 200 nmol/l to exceed 550 nmol/l. The impaired response is consistent with primary, secondary or tertiary **adrenal insufficiency** or steroid therapy. In Cushing's disease clearly the cortisol should be high.

In the long Synacthen® test, primary adrenal failure will show no response. Adrenals, however, that have been deprived of their stimulus for a long period of time, either due to pituitary or hypothalamic failure or due to suppression by exogenous steroids, will show a delayed response.

Answers – Data Interpretation 12 (5 marks)

1. B Renal tubular acidosis Type I
2. A Plain abdominal radiograph

The patient is unable to acidify his urine after an acid load. This is combined with a metabolic acidosis and a paradox hypokalaemia. The features are of **renal tubular acidosis Type I**. It is a defect of proton excretion in the distal tubule as opposed to proximal bicarbonate wastage in RTA Type II. In Type II the urine shows a normal depression of pH <5.4 in the ammonium chloride test.

There is a high incidence of renal stones and a sensitive way of detecting these is with the plain X-ray.

Answers – Data Interpretation 13 (5 marks)

1. C Polyglandular failure (Schmidt's syndrome)
2. A Auto-antibody screen

The serum electrolytes and the low morning cortisol indicate adreno-cortical insufficiency. In addition, the patient has features of hypothyroidism. The normal growth hormone and high TSH are against panhypopituitarism. **Polyglandular failure** is also associated with diabetes mellitus, pernicious anaemia, gonadal failure and hypo-parathyroidism. Hyperthyroidism may be seen if the auto-antibodies are of a stimulating kind. In the majority of patients, antibodies to the affected glandular tissue are found.

Answers – Data Interpretation 14 (6 marks)

1.
Best answers: **Chest X-ray/ACTH levels**
Accepted answers: CT thorax/Dexamethasone test
Rejected answer: Muscle biopsy

2.
Best answers: **Steroid myopathy/hypokalaemia**
Accepted answer: Paraneoplastic/Polymyositis/Eaton-Lambert syndrome
Rejected answers: Myasthenia gravis/Motor neurone disease

Neoplastic excretion of ectopic ACTH usually occurs with small cell carcinoma of the bronchus. Plasma cortisols are very high, the circadian rhythm is lost and there is no suppression with dexamethasone. This produces myopathy, diabetes mellitus, skin pigmentation, hyper-kalaemia and secondary alkalosis. The hoarse voice indicates recurrent laryngeal nerve palsy and inoperability.

The weakness in Eaton-Lambert syndrome is due to impaired release of acetylcholine and *improves* with exercise.

Answers – Data Interpretation 15 (5 marks)

1. D Polycystic ovary syndrome
2. C Ultrasound scan pelvis

PCO (Stein-Leventhal) syndrome is a syndrome of secondary virilization of genetically normal women. A spectrum of signs is found, the most prominent being hirsutism, menstrual irregularities and primary or secondary (!) infertility. The patients are frequently obese and, on ultrasound the ovaries are enlarged with multiple cysts. Serum testosterone is frequently elevated, as is the LH to FSH ratio (>3).

Although the ultrasound scan is very suggestive, cystic ovarial changes can also be seen in the other main differentials which are congenital adrenal hyperplasia and Cushing's syndrome. In the case given, the U&E's are against hypercortisolism and the normal hydroxyprogesterone is against congenital adrenal hyperplasia.

Patients with testicular feminisation never have periods as genetically they are men.

Answers – Data Interpretation 16 (5 marks)

1. A Hypogonadotrophic hypogonadism
2. C Craniopharyngioma

The patient has low gonadotrophins which show a delayed response to GN-RH. This indicates a functioning but chronically under-stimulated pituitary in keeping with a hypothalamic syndrome. In addition, the patient is hyperosmolar (plasma osmolality 305 mosmol/kg) in the presence of dilute urine, suggesting associated diabetes insipidus.

The combination of adiposity, central diabetes insipidus, hypogonadism and dwarfism has also been termed as 'dystrophy adiposo-genitalis' and is part of a syndrome caused by a **craniopharyngioma**. This benign tumour of Rathke's pouch can cause variable symptoms of pituitary compression or hypothalamic dysfunction. 15% occur within the pituitary fossa, they usually manifest themselves after the sixth year, but up to 50% remain asymptomatic until the third decade.

The patient may also present with headaches, bi-temporal hemianopia and suprasellar calcification on radiographs/CT. Besides hormone replacement, the patients frequently require surgery as the tumour is not radio-sensitive.

GASTROENTEROLOGY ANSWERS: CASE HISTORIES

Answers – Case History 1 (8 marks)

1. A Normal vitamin B_{12} metabolism

Both phases of the test are normal. The Dicopac® test combines the two phases of the Schilling test in one injection, the B_{12} and the B_{12}/intrinsic factor compound being labelled with different radioactive markers. Either phase of the test is abnormal if urinary excretion is less than 8%. Correction with intrinsic factor indicates pernicious anaemia.

2. B Candida

The described appearances are typical of Candidiasis. Herpes simplex being the main differential. However, this is less common and less likely to be so extensive. CMV typically causes giant ulcers.

3. C HIV infection

The combination of watery diarrhoea, normal FOBs, normal Dicopac® test and a submucosal process in the terminal ilium speak against Crohn's disease.

4. E Secondary lymphoma

Usually non-Hodgkin's lymphoma. It can affect any site including small bowel and brain.

The features of watery diarrhoea, normal Dicopac® test and a **sub**mucosal process exclude Crohn's disease. Lymphoma, TB and possibly Yersiniosis, remain differentials. **AIDS**-defining diseases include Kaposi's sarcoma (can occur anywhere in the body), oesophageal candida, PC-pneumonia, cerebral toxoplasmosis, CMV retinitis, recurrent Salmonella septicaemia, disseminated mycobacterial disease, non-Hodgkin's lymphoma, primary cerebral lymphoma and disseminated histoplasmosis (AIDS-defining equals any of the above with evidence of HIV infection).

Answers – Case History 2 (6 marks)

1. C Blood cultures and urine serology

The patient has a severe infectious disease, characterised by high fever, diarrhoea and hepatorenal failure with coagulopathy. Although abdominal ultrasound is sensible and a brain scan should be considered, liver biopsy and lumbar puncture would be contraindicated.

2. A Leptospirosis

The occupational history should alert to the possibility of Leptospiral infection.

Leptospirosis or **Weil's disease**, is caused by the spirochaete leptospira icterohaemorrhagiae. It is usually seen in patient groups that have a high exposure to animals and their urine, particularly rodents. Most common in veterinarians, abattoir workers and farmers, it is also found in sewage workers. Often taking a benign, self-limiting course, onset can be brutal with severe cardiovascular collapse. Generalised myalgia is typical, Serology is positive in blood and urine. Cultures from blood or CSF are only positive in first ten days. Severe hepatitis and renal failure may ensue. Antibiotic treatment is only rewarding if given within the first five days.

Answers – Case History 3 (8 marks)

1. A Endoscopy and small bowel biopsy

2. E Coeliac disease

This is a hypersensitivity to gluten, the protein contained in cereals. It is characterised by (subtotal) villous atrophy of the small bowel resulting in malabsorption. Symptoms are slow in onset and can present late in life usually with malaise and abdominal symptoms. Diarrhoea, recurrent stomatitis and sequelae of malabsorption i.e. osteomalacia, polyneuropathy and macrocytic anaemia are seen. Patients frequently show eosinophilia. Antigliadin and anti-reticulin antibodies are found in the majority of patients but can be normal. It is associated with dermatitis herpetiformis, an intensely itchy polymorphic skin rash. 10–20% show a familial incidence with variable expression.

3. C Poor diet

The condition usually responds to a gluten free diet, with the risk of relapse as the patient becomes asymptomatic.

4. B Small bowel carcinoma

There is an associated risk of small bowel malignancy, the risk of developing small bowel lymphoma is greatly reduced by a strict diet, as indicated in the history. However, the risk of developing small bowel carcinoma is not affected by avoidance of gluten, making this the more likely cause in this context.

Answers – Case History 4 (9 marks)

1.
Best answer: **Sclerosing cholangitis**
Accepted answers: Biliary obstruction/Bile ducts stones
Rejected answers: Hepatitis/Liver metastases/Hepatitis

The patient has clinical and biochemical features of obstructive jaundice. Up to 50% of **'primary' sclerosing cholangitides** are associated with inflammatory bowel disease, particularly ulcerative colitis.

2.
Best answer: **Ultrasound abdomen**
Accepted answers: ERCP/CT abdomen
Rejected answers: Hepatitis serology/Liver biopsy

3.
Best answer: **Nodal metastases from bowel carcinoma**
Accepted answers: Liver metastases/Lymphoma/Mirizzi syndrome
Rejected answers: Cholangiocarcinoma/Carcinoma of pancreas/Toxic megacolon

4.
Best answer: **Contrast enhanced CT abdomen**
Accepted answers: CT abdomen/Ultrasound abdomen/Colonoscopy
Rejected answers: ERCP/Liver biopsy

In addition the findings are suspicious of an extrinsic compression of the bile duct at the porta hepatis. This is most likely due to a nodal mass. With a history of active ulcerative colitis greater than ten years, a metastasized carcinoma of the colon has to be considered. The CT would assess the large bowel as well as the liver and the extrahepatic bile duct. Other complications of ulcerative colitis include amyloid, sero-negative arthritis, Erythema nodosum, Pyoderma gangrenosum and uveitis and episcleritis. Fistulae, and abscesses are a feature of Crohn's disease due to the transmural inflammation of the bowel.

Answers – Case History 5 (8 marks)

1.
Best answers: **Urinary porphyrins/Abdominal ultrasound**
Accepted answers: Hepatitis serology/Chest X-ray/Water deprivation test
Rejected answers: Liver biopsy/Psychiatric assessment
2.
Best answer: **Acute intermittent porphyria**
Accepted answers: Porphyria/Chronic hepatitis
Rejected answers: Psychogenic polydipsia

3.
Best answer: **Stop fluoxetine**
Accepted answers: Avoid alcohol/Drug counselling

A combination of a low serum osmolality and a high urine osmolality indicates inappropriate ADH secretion. Causes for this include any intracranial pathology (tumour/abscess/increased pressure), intrathoracic pathology (infection, in particular legionella, empyema, tumour), drugs (promazine, carbamazepine, chlopropramide), lymphoma and acute porphyrias.

A triad of recurrent episodes of peritonism, neuro-psychiatric disturbances and hyponatraemia is typical for **acute intermittent porphyria**. Urine turns orange/brown on standing and there is a familial incidence (autosomal dominant). It is precipitated by a number of drugs, in particular alcohol, oral contraceptives, anti-depressants, barbiturates, benzodiazopines and a number of antibiotics (for full list, see BNF). If the syndrome is combined with a photosensitive rash, this indicates the much rarer variegate porphyria, which is more common in white South Africans.

Answer – Case History 6 (10 marks)

1. X-linked recessive inheritance

2.
Best answer: **Right psoas haematoma**
Accepted answers: Psoas haematoma/Retroperitoneal haemorrhage/ Psoas abscess
Rejected answers: Renal haematoma/Renal abscess/Intra-articular haemorrhage of right hip

The combination of flank pain and inability to extend the hip indicates irritation of the psoas muscle, a common site for haemorrhage.

3.
Best answer: **Chronic Hepatitis C with cirrhosis**
Accepted answers: Transfusion cirrhosis/Chronic Hepatitis C
Rejected answers: Liver failure/Auto-immune hepatitis/Hepatitis B

The patient has additional evidence of liver failure, with deranged LFTs and a raised INR. The deficiency of factor VIII does not affect the extrinsic pathway of the clotting cascade. The raised INR indicates established liver damage. Up to 20% of patients with **Hepatitis C** develop cirrhosis.

4.
Best answers: **Liver ultrasound/Hepatitis serology**
Accepted answers: Liver biopsy after correction of clotting/Gastroscopy to exclude varices
Rejected answers: Liver biopsy/CT abdomen

Although a liver biopsy is desirable in a patient with chronic hepatitis, a non-invasive method has to be chosen in the first instance. The young age of the patient is against Hepatitis B, as serological tests for blood components were available in the 1980's.

Answers – Case History 7 (10 marks)

1. B Stool microscopy and culture

The acute onset of two family members suggests **food poisoning**. Most of these have an incubation period of less than one week, indicating a source other than traveller's diarrhoea. The commonest pathogens would be *E. coli*, Salmonella, Shigella and Staphylococcus. Campylobacter and viral infection may also have to be considered.

2. E Erythema nodosum

Painful red to purple nodules erupt over the extensor surfaces of the upper and lower limbs. In 50% this is idiopathic. It is associated with granulomatous diseases (TB, Sarcoid, Leprosy), inflammatory bowel disease, infections (Streptococcus, Salmonella, Yersinia) and a number of drugs (penicillin, sulphonamides, OCP).

3. A X-ray of both wrists and pelvis

4. C Reiter's syndrome

The patient has developed an asymmetrical polyarthritis of large joints, probably associated with a sacro-ileitis. Breathlessness may be due to associated pericarditis or pleuritis/pleural effusion. Other features include uveitis, Keratoderma blenorrhagica (an exfoliative process of palms and soles), and a circinate balanitis (a well demarcated rash of the glans of the penis). The latter two are more common in **Reiter's syndrome** following non-specific urethritis.

Septic arthritis may occur after some earlier infection, but would be most unusual to be polyarticular. Immune complex vasculitis (Type III hypersensitivity) may be observed after chronic low grade infection. There is no specific test for Reiter's disease. If severe, characteristic X-ray changes with erosions and a fluffy periostial reaction may be seen.

5. A Non-steroidal anti-inflammatory drugs

Treatment is symptomatic.

Answers – Case History 8 (10 marks)

1.
Best answers: **Blood glucose/Liver ultrasound/Liver function tests/Serum ferritin**
Accepted answers: Liver biopsy/HbA1c
Rejected answers: Rheumatoid factor/Autoimmune screen

2.
Best answer: **Haemochromatosis**
Accepted answer: Wilson's disease
Rejected answers: Chronic active hepatitis/Rheumatoid arthitis

The patient has the key features skin pigmentation, hepatomegaly, degenerative joint disease and features of diabetes mellitus. **Haemochromatosis** is an inherited disease characterised by excessive iron deposition throughout the body. This is exacerbated by excess alcohol intake. Expression is milder in women due to the menstrual blood loss.

3.
Best answer: **Liver biopsy for dry iron content**
Accepted answers: Liver biopsy/Ferritin levels
Rejected answer: Bone marrow biopsy

An iron stain (i.e. Pearl's) will demonstrate the increased iron content in the liver (which incidentally is also seen on MR scanning).

4.
Best answer: **Autosomal recessive inheritance**
Accepted answer: Recessive family trait

Most inborn errors of metabolism are autosomal recessive. This pattern of inheritance is characterised by the fact that not every generation is affected and that male to male transmission occurs.

5.
Best answer: **Hepatocellular carcinoma**
Accepted answer: Liver cirrhosis
Rejected answer: HCC

Up to one-third of patients with liver cirrhosis progress to development of hepatoma. The presence of cirrhosis in this patient is indicated by the reduction in hepatic size and splenomegaly. (HCC is rejected as this is an uncommon abbreviation.)

GASTROENTEROLOGY ANSWERS: DATA INTERPRETATIONS

Answers – Data Interpretation 1 (5 marks)

1. C Acquired hypogammaglobinaemia
2. D Chronic giardia infection

There is isolated reduction of all the immunoglobulins. The age of the patient is against Hodgkin disease, normal clinical examination and normal full blood count make Non-Hodgkin's lymphoma unlikely and exclude yellow nail syndrome. Recurrent infections are the main manifestations of **acquired hypogammaglobulinaemia**. Causes for diarrhoea are bacterial overgrowth and chronic infections, in particular giardia. An inflammatory colitis may occur.

Answers – Data Interpretation 2 (6 marks)

1. C Gilbert's syndrome
2. A Autosomal dominant
3. E Nicotinic acid test

The hereditary hyperbilirubinaemias are characterised by an increase in unconjugated bilirubin (G**i**lbert's and Cr**i**gler-Najjar = **i**nconjugated) and c**o**njugated bilirubin (Dubin-Johns**o**n and R**o**tor). Conjugated bilirubin is water soluble and is excreted in the urine, these two are excluded by the normal dipstix. **Gilbert's syndrome** has an excellent prognosis and is often discovered incidentally. It is characterised by a mild elevation of bilirubin which shows a slow rise in the nicotinic acid test, with a high and delayed peak at 2–3 hours (usually around 40–60 μmol/l). Peak levels in normal individuals are reached at 90 minutes (usually less than 25 μmol/l). An increase in bilirubin is also provoked by three days fasting (less than 400 kcal/day).

Answers – Data Interpretation 3 (4 marks)

1. E Anti-mitochondrial antibodies
2. C Primary biliary cirrhosis

A middle-aged woman presents with generalised pruritus, steatorrhoea and evidence of sicca syndrome. Her globulins are elevated (markedly raised IgM).

PBC is a chronic, aseptic distructive cholangitis. It accounts for approximately 1% of liver cirrhosis. 90% are of women in their fifth decade. Pruritus precedes jaundice, biliary obstruction leads to maldigestion. It is associated with Sjögren's syndrome, polyarthralgia, autoimmune thyroiditis and hypercholesterolaemia. Antimitochondrial antibodies are found in over 90%, of the several subtypes Anti-M_2 are specific. Titres are elevated above 1:100.

Answers – Data Interpretation 4 (4 marks)

1. B Zieve syndrome
2. E Spurious hyponatraemia

The patient has a combination of hypercholesterolaemia and haemolytic anaemia as indicated by the increased reticulocyte count (greater than 2%) and increased unconjugated bilirubin. Haptoglobin estimation would show this to be reduced. On the social background given, alcoholism has to be assumed, the triad of these features is termed **Zieve syndrome** (alcoholism, hypercholesterolaemia and haemolytic anaemia). Sodium that low indicates that the patient is either very ill, or that there has been error in the estimation. In hyperlipidaemia the sodium is only contained within the aqueous phase of the blood sample, whilst the blood sample volume is increased by the lipid phase giving a falsely low reading. Hyperaldosteronism secondary to liver cirrhosis may contribute, but is unlikely to produce levels this low.

Answers – Data Interpretation 5 (6 marks)

1. B Autoimmune chronic active hepatitis
2. C Hepatitis serology
3. A Azathioprine

Autoimmune CAH in women typically presents with malaise, tender hepatomegaly, secondary amenorrhoea and elevated LFTs. Without immune suppressant therapy, prognosis is bad, however with therapy ten year survival rate is usually higher than 90%. Non-specific manifestations of chronic liver disease are found. The disease may be complicated by development of hepatocellular carcinoma.

Answers – Data Interpretation 6 (6 marks)

1.

Best answer: **Chronic pancreatitis**
Accepted answers: Pancreatitis/Maldigestion
Rejected answers: Malabsorption/Acute pancreatitis

2.

Best answers: **Chronic alcohol abuse/Gallstones/Bile duct stones**
Accepted answers: Hypercalcaemia/Hyperlipidaemia/Haemochromatosis
Rejected answers: Crohn's disease/Whipple's disease/Coeliac disease

3.

Best answers: **Abdominal X-ray/Abdominal ultrasound/ERCP**
Accepted answers: Amylase/CT abdomen/Pancreatic function test
Rejected answers: Gastroscopy/Small bowel biopsy/Small bowel enema

Faecal fat excretion is high (> 30 g in 3 days) but xylose absorption and excretion is normal. This excludes malabsorption and small bowel cause for steatorrhoea. The most likely cause is chronic pancreatitis either due to gallstones or alcohol. Other causes include haemochromatosis, hyperlipidaemia, primary biliary sclerosis and sclerosing cholangitis.

Answers – Data Interpretation 7 (4 marks)

1.

Best answers: **Blind loop syndrome/Bacterial overgrowth**
Accepted answers: Short bowel syndrome/Anastomotic carcinoma
Rejected answer: Zollinger-Ellison syndrome/Dumping syndrome

2.

Best answers: **Small bowel aspiration culture/Radiocarbon breath test/Hydrogen breath test**
Accepted answers: Schilling test pre and post antibiotics
Rejected answers: Endoscopy/Barium follow through

The likely treatment for ulcers at that time would have been a partial gastrectomy either with anterograde anastomosis between the stomach and the duodenum (Billroth 1 gastrectomy) or a side-to-side anastomosis with the jejunum (Billroth 2 or Polya gastroenterostomy). The delayed onset of the symptoms is against dumping syndrome, this is excluded by the normal oral glucose tolerance test (dumping syndrome should show a sharp drop in the one hour value to hypoglycaemic levels). The macrocytic anaemia suggests bacterial overgrowth in a blind ending afferent loop. This could be confirmed by endoscopy and aspiration or a hydrogen or radiocarbon breath test (increased bacterial activity breaks down the radioactive compound leading to increased excretion of radioactive gas through the lungs).

Answers – Data Interpretation 8 (5 marks)

1. C Whipple's disease
2. D Polymerase chain reaction from duodenal biopsy

Whipple's disease is caused by *Tropheryma Whippelii*, a bacterium that can be identified within macrophages under the electron microscope. The identification of PAS positive glycoproteins within macrophages in the lamina propria of the small bowel is diagnostic, however PCR techniques will allow direct identification of the rod. Typically affecting middle-aged men, it presents with diarrhoea, abdominal pain and malabsorption. Extra intestinal manifestations include fever, polyarthritis, polyserositis, lymphadenopathy and skin pigmentation. Therapy is with prolonged (3–6 months) antibiotics (i.e. tetracycline).

Answers – Data Interpretation 9 (6 marks)

1. E Budd-Chiari syndrome
2. A Prolonged severe illness in the neonatal period
3. C Fundal varices

Budd-Chiari syndrome or hepatic vein thrombosis is seen in the context of thrombophilia, red cell anomalies and severe illnesses associated with chronic sepsis and dehydration. It results in post-hepatic portal hypertension with consecutive liver damage. The caudate lobe (segment one) is usually spared as this has separate portal and arterial supply as well as venous drainage. It results in compensatory hypertrophy of this lobe. The ascites seen in this context is frequently an exudate rather than a transudate, however the normal glucose essentially rules out infection. Fundal varices will not be treated by sclerotherapy of the oesophagus alone. Umbilical vein catheters cause portal vein thrombosis.

Answers: Data Interpretation 10 (5 marks)

1. A HELLP syndrome
2. E Delivery of baby

Pre-eclampsia is defined as hypertension developing in the last three months of pregnancy, with associated oedema and proteinuria. The aim is to control the blood pressure. Whereas eclampsia is characterised by hypertension, proteinuria, oedema, coagulopathy and focal necrosis of the liver, **HELLP** is defined as the syndrome of the **H**aemolysis **E**levated **L**FTs and **L**ow **P**latelets. Either condition requires urgent delivery.

Acute fatty liver of pregnancy occurs after thirty weeks. It consists of acute fatty degeneration of the liver, hepato renal failure, DIC and encephalopathy. It resolves with delivery. Cholestasis (intra-hepatic) of pregnancy also occurs in the third trimester and presents with pruritus, jaundice and may lead to premature labour and post-partum haemorrhage. It also resolves spontaneously within two weeks after delivery.

Answers – Data Interpretation 11 (6 marks)

1.
Best answer: **Therapy with proton pump inhibitor**
Accepted answers: Gastrectomy/Atrophic gastritis/Antacid therapy
Rejected answer: Zollinger-Ellison syndrome

2.
Best answers: **Chronic atrophic gastritis/Helicobacter gastritis**
Accepted answer: Pernicious anaemia
Rejected answer: Previous partial gastrectomy

3.
Best answer: **Gastroscopy and urease test**
Accepted answer: Helicobacter serology
Rejected answer: Contrast enhanced CT pancreas

Causes for elevated gastrin levels include ZES, atrophic gastritis, pernicious anaemia, Helicobacter gastritis, previous antrectomy and therapy with proton pump inhibitors. However, pernicious anaemia does not present with relapsing ulcers and the patient has not had previous surgery. ZES is characterised by a paradoxical *increase* of gastrin after administration of secretin, by at least 100%.

Answers – Data Interpretation 12 (5 marks)

1. E Hydatid disease
2. E CT brain

The history suggests a rupture of **hydatid liver cyst**, as indicated by an allergic reaction, fever and bilirubinuria. Cerebral hydatid cysts have to be excluded in view of the fit.

Answers – Data Interpretation 13 (5 marks)

1. D Insulinoma
2. D CT pancreas

On one occasion the patient shows morning hypoglycaemia, on a further morning hyperglycaemia, the latter likely to be due to rebound phenomenon (Somogyi effect) or the patient having eaten to combat the hypoglycaemia in the early hours. The raised C-peptide after a fast indicates there is inappropriate insulin secretion. Factitious insulin administration would not result in elevation of the C-peptide, which is produced by cleavage from endogenous pro-insulin. Most insulinomas tumours are benign, they are however frequently seen as part of Multiple Endocrine Neoplasia Type I (pancreatic tumours, parathyroid hyperplasia and medullary carcinoma of the thyroid).

Answers – Data Interpretation 14 (5 marks)

1. B Pseudomyxoma peritonei
2. D Krukenberg metastases

Gelatinous ascites is seen with **mucinous adenocarcinomas** of the ovary and GI tract. The past history suggests intra-peritoneal metastases (Krukenberg metastases). These spread through the pouch of Douglas to the ovaries following gravity.

Answers – Data Interpretation 15 (6 marks)

1. B Abdominal ultrasound
2. A Streptococcal liver abscess
3. E Percutaneous drainage

The patient has features of chronic sepsis with a normocytic anaemia, low albumin, raised globulins, raised ESR and intermittent pyrexia. This is localised to the right upper quadrant. The history of left iliac fossa irritation is suggestive of either diverticular disease/diverticulitis or carcinoma of the colon. The most likely diagnosis is a **streptococcus milleri abscess** which accounts for over 75% of liver abscesses. Most of these are secondary to a predisposing cause relating to the GI tract.

Answers – Data Interpretation 16 (6 marks)

1.
Best answer: **Lag storage curve**
Accepted answer: Delayed hypoglycaemia
Rejected answer: Diabetes mellitus

2.
Best answer: **Wilson's disease**
Accepted answer: Drug abuse
Rejected answer: Haemochromatosis

3.
Best answer: **Coeruloplasmin levels**
Accepted answers: Liver biopsy/Urine copper after penicillamine
Rejected answer: CT brain

Lag storage curves are also seen in renal failure, gastrectomy and some normal patients. **Wilson's disease** (hepato-lenticular degeneration) is an autosomal recessive defect of copper excretion. Coeruloplasmin, the serum transport and storage protein is markedly reduced. Biliary excretion of copper is impaired leading to increased renal excretion and deposition of copper throughout the body. Deposition in liver, CNS, Cornea (Kayser-Fleischer ring), renal failure/type 2 renal tubular acidosis, cardiomyopathy and haemolytic anaemia can be seen. Renal excretion is increased with the chelating agent D-penicillamine, which is the therapy of choice.

HAEMATOLOGY ANSWERS: CASE HISTORIES

Answers – Case History 1 (9 marks)

1. B Erythrocyte sedimentation rate
2. E Prothrombin time
3. C Venesection
4. D Myelofibrosis

A middle-aged patient with an increase in all cell lines and splenomegaly. The combination of polycythaemia and iron depletion indicates **polycythaemia rubra vera**.

This is a myeloprofilerative disorder with a peak incidence in the sixth decade, men commoner than women. Endogenous erythropoietin is reduced distinguishing it from secondary polycythaemia, causes for which include chronic airways disease, stress polycythaemia (Gaissböck syndrome) and EPO-secreting tumours (hepatoma, hypernephroma and cerebellar haemangioblastoma). Alkaline leucocyte phosphatase (ALP) is elevated in contrast to CML. Although platelets may be increased, platelet function is often reduced with a tendency for bruising and an increased bleeding time. The increased cell turnover may precipitate gout.

Therapy in the first instance is with venaesection in order to keep the haematocrit below 45%. Second line treatment includes 5-hydroxyurea, but with an increased risk of secondary leukaemia.

Complications: embolism (stroke and PE accounting for up to 40% of deaths), haemorrhage, myelofibrosis and acute leukaemia. The latter occurs in under 2% when treated with venaesection and up to 10–15% under myelo-suppressive chemotherapy.

As a late feature, the patient develops a leuco-erythroblastic blood film with left shift of all cell lines, indicating extra-medullary erythropoiesis.

Answers – Case History 2 (9 marks)

1. C Blood cultures and standard blood film
2. A Resuscitation and iv penicillin
3. B Pneumococcal vaccination
4. E Viral infection

A young coloured patient with a suspicious deficit in family history (Cave – the adopted child!) presents with features of a lobar pneumonia. In addition, he has a macrocytic anaemia (reticulocytosis) with changes in the skeleton. In combination, the features suggest **sickle cell crisis** complicated/precipitated by pneumococcal pneumonia. Treatment is with aggressive rehydration, analgesia and antibiotics suitable for the organism as well as the patient (child!).

As homozygous patients with sickle cell disease will develop splenic atrophy due to infarction, pneumococcal vaccination is mandatory. Hyposplenism is evident on re-admission due to the presence of Howell-Jolly bodies (nuclear residues within erythrocytes).

Infection with Parvovirus B19 (fifth disease, slapped cheek disease) which otherwise is a benign self-limiting viral infection can lead to aplastic crisis in patients with haemolytic anaemias.
Other complications include infarction of other organs, in particular bone and the development of *Salmonella osteomyelitis*.

Diagnosis is by blood film and haemoglobin electrophoresis which shows replacement of glutamine by valine in the beta chain. Homozygous patients will have approximately 80% HbS and 20% HbF.

Answers – Case History 3 (9 marks)

1. C Blood film
2. E α-interferon
3. B Renal vein thrombosis
4. C Essential thrombocythaemia

The patient has dramatic elevation of the platelet count with mild associated leucocytosis. In addition, he has a microcytic anaemia which may either be due to chronic GI blood loss or depletion of iron stores by associated polycythaemia. The patient has a raised urate indicating increased cell turnover. Thrombocytosis to this degree is highly suggestive of **essential thrombocythaemia** which has an association (up to 30%) of gastro-duodenal ulceration. Philadelphia chromosome is absent, and the ALP is increased (DD:CML). The blood film shows megakaryocytes, the diagnosis can be confirmed by marrow biopsy. Complications include thromboembolism (main cause of death), haemorrhage (deficit in platelet function) and transformation to acute leukaemia (10%). The patients affected are usually over 50 years, mean survival time 10 to 15 years.

Therapy is successful in the majority of cases with α-interferon, second line is myelo-suppressant therapy (5-hydroxyurea). In acute thrombotic crises, thrombocytapheresis may be required. Anti-platelet drugs are contra-indicated.

Answers – Case History 4 (10 marks)

1. D Anti-phospholipid antibodies
2. B Auto-immune haemolytic anaemia
3. E Auto-antibody screen
4. A Retinal vein branch occlusion
5. B Aspirin

A young woman has recurrent thromboses. This suggests a hyper-coagulable state but may also be due to a red cell defect (HbC, HbS) or an increase in red cells or platelets.

The APTT, however, shows a paradoxical prolongation which does not correct after addition of normal plasma. This suggests an active inhibiting factor, such as anti-phospholipid antibodies. The antibodies interfere with the test giving a false result. In addition, the patient has evidence of an auto-immune haemolytic anaemia with a positive Coombs' test (the red cells are laden with auto-antibodies) and a compensatory reticulocytosis.

Subsequently, the patient developed renal impairment and hypertension. The patient has **systemic lupus erythematodes**.

Venous occlusion and haemorrhage has occurred in the eye, arterial occlusion would lead to a pale (anaemic) area in the fundus. Long-standing significant hypertension is excluded by the absence of hypertensive changes. The treatment for this is aspirin, more aggressive anti-coagulation will exacerbate the retinal haemorrhage.

Answers – Case History 5 (7 marks)

1. A Thrombin time
2. D Anti-thrombin III deficiency
3. D Heparin side-effect

A young patient presents with features of thrombophilia. Despite full heparinisation, the patient develops a further thrombosis. The resistance to heparin therapy is characteristic of **anti-thrombin III deficiency**.

Anti-thrombin III is an inhibitor of clotting factors mainly directed against the activity of thrombin, Factor Xa and Factor IXa and other clotting factors. It is the mediator of the effect of heparin, in the presence of which it is an effective inhibitor of thrombin and Factor Xa. There is a spectrum of congenital AT III-deficiencies which vary in the levels of AT III as well as its activity. The commonest form is transmitted as an autosomal dominant trait. The main differentials being protein C and protein S deficiency.

An important side-effect of heparin is the induction of thrombocytopenia and the BNF (Edition 38) recommends monitoring of platelet levels for patients on heparin for longer than five days.

Answers – Case History 6 (9 marks)

1.
Best answer: **Bone marrow biopsy**
Accepted answers: Haematinics/Lead levels
Rejected answers: Ultrasound of abdomen/Staging CT

2.
Best answer: **Myelo-dysplastic syndrome**
Accepted answers: Aplastic anaemia/sideroblastic anaemia
Rejected answers: Lymphoma/CML/CLL

3.
Best answer: **Invasive aspergillosis**
Accepted answers: Aspergillosis/Tuberculosis
Rejected answers: Mycetoma/ABPA/Squamous lung carcinoma

4.
Best answer: **Acute myeloid leukaemia**
Accepted answer: Malignant transformation
Rejected answers: CML/Lymphoma

The patient has a bi-cytopaenia with an excess of blasts and the presence of ring sideroblasts. This indicates a **myelo-dysplastic syndrome** (FAB classification **RAEB**, refractory anaemia with excess of blasts). However, the diagnosis of MDS requires exclusion of leukaemia and aplastic syndromes and more benign conditions, such as B_{12} or folate deficiency, drug induced and post-infectious marrow suppression. Therapy is supportive, good results have been achieved with stimulators of haemopoiesis, such as erythropoietin and GM-CSF. CMML is one end of the spectrum of MDS. MDS can transform into acute myeloid leukaemia or acute myelo-monocytic leukaemia. The latter is a further cause of gingiva (gum) hyperplasia (besides phenytoin).

Invasive aspergillosis, a cavitating infection can occur in any form of immune-compromise. This has to be distinguished from mycetoma, which is a fungus ball in a pre-existing cavity and from allergic bronchial pulmonary aspergillosis which is a hypersensitivity reaction to the ubiquitous fungus. This typically occurs in young asthmatic men. ABPA leads to proximal bronchiectases.

Answers – Case History 7 (7 marks)

1. C Angiodysplasia
2. A Right hemicolectomy

The patient has a microcytic anaemia with a history of blood loss. The normal barium enema in combination with the abnormal angiogram suggests **angiodysplasia of the colon**. Angiodysplasia is a common finding and it can be difficult to decide whether it is responsible for a GI bleed. Acute haemorrhage may be controlled by embolisation, but this carries a risk of bowel necrosis. Treatment is usually by resection.

3. D Benign monoclonal gammopathy

The most important differential diagnosis is multiple myeloma. However, the normal calcium, alk. phosphatase, renal function and, in particular, low levels of bone marrow plasma cells (< 10%) are against myeloma, although this is not entirely excluded. Further investigations would require a more detailed investigation of the gamma band and a skeletal survey.

HAEMATOLOGY ANSWERS: DATA INTERPRETATIONS

Answers – Data Interpretation 1 (6 marks)

1. C Bone marrow biopsy
2. B Hodgkin disease
3. D iv antibiotics

A young patient with no obvious precipitating cause for a profound pancytopaenia. The most important and probably most likely cause is an **acute leukaemia with an aleukaemic blood film** (no blasts). The patient has evidence of sepsis in the presence of absolute granulocytopaenia and requires immediate covering with broad spectrum antibiotics.

Hodgkin disease presents with lymphadenopathy, usually in the mediastinum. Severe bone marrow infiltration would be evident by a leuco-erythroblastic blood film.

Answers – Data Interpretation 2 (6 marks)

1. A Bleeding time
2. D Symptomatic therapy only
3. D Autosomal dominant

A young boy has a bleeding disorder suggestive of platelet dysfunction. The platelet count is normal ruling out idiopathic thrombocytopenic purpura. The associated regenerating anaemia is most likely due to the previous surgery.

Haemophilia is excluded as the patient, being male, would be homozygous (X-linked recessive) and the clotting results would be markedly abnormal. In addition, petechial haemorrhages indicate a platelet problem.

There is a mild reduction in Factor VIII concentration which, on its own, is unlikely to be symptomatic (concentrations over 50% are usually not clinically important). However, the combination of platelet dysfunction and mild Factor VIII reduction indicates **von Willebrand syndrome**. This autosomal dominant condition (variable penetrance) is characterised by a deficiency in the large molecular fraction of Factor VIII (F VIII vWF) which is responsible for platelet aggregation. The bleeding time is prolonged and diagnosis is made by Factor VIII vWF assay.

Answers – Data Interpretation 3 (6 marks)

1.
Best answer: **Sickle cell trait**
Rejected answer: Sickle cell disease

2.
Best answer: **Beta-thalassaemia minor**
Accepted answer: Beta-thalassaemia
Rejected answer: Thalassaemia/haemoglobin C disease

3. 1:4/25% (Sickle-beta thalassaemia)

A women with haemoglobin S who remains asymptomatic into the first trimester must be heterozygous. In the homozygous form, HbS is greater than 90%.

The father has a mild anaemia, but no reduction in red cells and a severe microcytosis. The presence of HbF ($\alpha_2\ \gamma_2$), and increased HbA_2 ($\alpha_2\ \delta_2$) over 5% indicates a problem with the β-chains. However, the haemoglobin being above 10 again indicates a heterozygous condition. The child has a 1:4 chance, each of the following constellations:

- Normal haemoglobin
- Sickle cell trait
- Beta-thalassaemia trait
- **Sickle beta-thalassaemia**

The first three conditions are not associated with serious problems (see parents), but the last configuration is a true sickling syndrome which, in its manifestations, can approach homozygous sickle cell disease.

Answers – Data Interpretation 4 (4 marks)

1. C D-dimer levels and blood cultures
2. B Amniotic fluid embolus

The patient has **disseminated intravascular coagulation** as evidenced by intravascular haemolysis (red cell fragmentation), thrombocytopenia and abnormal clotting, in particular the thrombin time indicating consumption of the clotting factors.

The most likely cause is an obstetric complication, however it would be unusual for infection to cause this degree of disease within such a short period of time, and the white cell count is relatively low for extensive septicaemia. Multiple tests are appropriate in this scenario, but D-dimer levels and blood cultures are the most sensible combination, as one test confirms the diagnosis whereas the other one excludes an important differential.

In DIC the thrombin time is prolonged by a) consumption of fibrinogen and b) the presence of FDP which interfere with the formation of cross-linked fibrin. This is partially corrected for by the addition of protamin sulphate, although this is not a test required to make the diagnosis.

There are many causes of DIC, the commonest being sepsis. In the young woman other causes would include abruptio placentae, septic abortion and toxic shock syndrome.

The most important step in the management is treatment of the underlying condition. Severe haemorrhage may require FFP.

Answers – Data Interpretation 5 (4 marks)

1.

Best answer: **Vitamin B_{12} deficiency/Vegetarianism**
Accepted answers: Folate deficiency/Alcohol induced
Rejected answers: Iron deficiency/Chronic blood loss/Pernicious anaemia

2.

Best answers: **Vitamin B_{12} levels/Blood film/Haematinics**
Accepted answers: Liver function tests/thyroid function tests
Rejected answers: Bone marrow biopsy/Schilling test

A macrocytic anaemia with mild reduction in white cell count and platelets in an Asian woman is most likely to be **nutritional**. Strict Hindu diet is free of animal produce. Other causes to be considered would be toxic, including alcohol and myelodysplasia, but these are much less likely. Pernicious anaemia is essentially excluded by the low gastrin.

First line investigations should confirm B_{12} deficiency before any more invasive procedures are performed.

Answers – Data Interpretation 6 (4 marks)

1. C Multiple myeloma
2. B ESR

The patient has several features of **myeloma**: osteoporosis with vertebral collapse, polyuria (hypercalcaemia), normochromic anaemia (and low white cells and platelets). None of these features are diagnostic, however the rouleaux formation on the blood film suggests an increase in blood protein.

A bone scan is not helpful for myeloma as this only assesses increased osteoblastic activity. Approximately two-thirds of patients with myeloma have Bence-Jones proteins (light chains) in their urine however a small proportion do not excrete abnormal protein. The anaemia is a poor prognostic factor and, in combination, with the hypercalcaemia makes Waldenström's very unlikely.

Tuberculous spondylitis typically affects more than one vertebral segment, is unlikely to cause the blood changes and would show up on the bone scan.

A raised ESR would not necessarily differentiate between infection, myeloma or metastatic disease.

Answers – Data Interpretation 7 (5 marks)

1. E Lead poisoning
2. A Abdominal X-ray

Lead intoxication is becoming rare since the withdrawal of lead-containing paints. However, neglected children especially may still present after chronic ingestion = pica syndrome (Lat. pica = magpie). Lead residue is well demonstrated on X-ray if still present within the bowel.

Pallor is caused by anaemia as well as vasospasm. Other features are lead-lines on the gums, constipation, neuropathy and encephalopathy. δ-amino-laevulanic acid is increased in blood and urine.

Differential of sideroblastic anaemia include hereditary causes, myeloproliferative disorders, toxins (lead, alcohol, anti-TB drugs), leukaemia and connective tissue diseases.

A di-morphic film indicates two erythrocyte populations of different ages such as seen after blood transfusion, treated iron deficiency, combined iron and B_{12} deficiency and sideroblastic anaemia.

Answers – Data Interpretation 8 (5 marks)

1. C Immune electrophoresis
2. C Cold haemagglutinin disease

The absence of a blanching phase preceding purple discoloration in the hands exposed to cold indicates that this is not true Raynaud's syndrome.
The patient has delayed haemolysis of one blood sample after cooling and re-warming. This is essentially the basis of the Donath-Landsteiner reaction which confirms the presence of cold haemagglutinins. These are found in **chronic cold haemagglutinin disease** where there are complement fixating monoclonal-antibodies of IgM class against red cells. It is a condition of the elderly which may precede lymphoma. Chronic haemolysis leads to pigment gallstones.

A similar picture is found following infection in children where it is called **paroxysmal cold haemoglobinuria**. It is seen in congenital syphilis and after viral infections, such as measles, mumps or chickenpox. The antibodies, however, are polyclonal IgG.

Answers – Data Interpretation 9 (4 marks)

1. C Hodgkin disease
2. A Radiotherapy

Hodgkin disease has two age peaks in the third and seventh decade and is more common in men. Presentation is with fever, weight loss, malaise, lymphadenopathy and/or hepatomegaly. Staging depends on the number of lymph stations and extralymphatic organs involved.

As far as can be said, the patient has no adenopathy and no evidence of hepatosplenomegaly. The commonest presentation is with mediastinal adenopathy (stage one). The treatment for stage one is radiotherapy, the prognosis is excellent.

Alcohol induced nodal pain is a rare but typical manifestation, as is an undulating fever (Pel-Ebstein fever).

Answers – Data Interpretation 10 (5 marks)

1. B Direct Coombs' test
2. C Delayed transfusion reaction

Delayed transfusion reactions occur in patients previously exposed to "foreign red cell antigens" such as previous transfusions or pregnancy. A positive direct Coombs' test will confirm that the transfused red cells are laden with antibodies. (An indirect Coombs' test only confirms the presence of free antibodies.)

The patient requires re-testing of her serum against standard red cells to identify the antibodies produced. Antibodies frequently exist against multiple epitopes. In addition, the patient needs to be re cross-matched against the units received which would also be useful for an estimate of how many of the units received are likely to have haemolysed.

Answers – Data Interpretation 11 (4 marks)

1. C Gold
2. D Blood film

In rheumatoid arthritis, all types of anaemia can be found. Most are **drug-induced**, but there are associated auto-immune conditions, such as pernicious anaemia and hypothyroidism and there is the anaemia of chronic disease and hypersplenism (Felty's syndrome).

Chronic GI bleed is found with non-steroidal anti-inflammatory drugs, methotrexate is a folate antagonist, sulphasalazine causes intravascular haemolysis with compensatory reticulocytosis which can raise the MCV.

Gold and D-penicillamine, however, cause aplastic anaemia.

Answers – Data Interpretation 12 (2 marks)

1. B Haemolysis

An old favourite!

The discrepancy lies between the fact that the patient is by definition reasonably well as he is an out-patient and the grossly abnormal biochemical profile which, if correct, suggests that the patient is probably unconscious, if not dead. The answer lies in **delayed**

processing of a sample which was left uncentrifuged on the shelf overnight and has haemolysed.

Answers – Data Interpretation 13 (6 marks)

1. B Discontinue any medication
2. A Glucose-6-phosphate-dehydrogenase deficiency
3. E X-linked recessive

G-6-PD deficiency (Favism) is world-wide the second most common inherited condition after diabetes mellitus. Haemolytic crises are precipitated by ingestion of white beans (Fava beans) most anti-malarial drugs (Kenya!), antibiotics (sulphonamides, nitrofurantoin, chloramphenicol), Vitamin K, aspirin and many others. Blood count and blood film are normal between attacks. During a crisis there is evidence of haemolysis (bite cells, Heinz bodies and reticulocytosis).

Diagnosis is by direct measurement of the enzyme levels. In a crisis any precipitating cause has to be removed, blood transfusions may be required in severe cases. Splenectomy is not indicated.

Answers – Data Interpretation 14 (4 marks)

1. C Red cell mass
2. B Stop smoking

The patient fulfils virtually all the criteria for **stress polycythaemia** (Gaissböck syndrome). He is a hypertensive smoker on diuretics with a relative increase in red cell volume. The absolute red cell mass is not increased which distinguishes it from polycythaemia rubra vera. Blood viscosity, however, is increased with the risk thrombo-embolic episodes. The most important factor is to stop smoking, venaesection may be required. Chronic hypoxia in a smoker will be evident in arterial blood gases and leads to secondary increase in erythropoietin. Carboxyhaemoglobin levels are increased up to 15% in smokers.

NEPHROLOGY ANSWERS: CASE HISTORIES

Answers – Case History 1 (9 marks)

1. E Hypernephroma
2. D Hyperreninaemia
3. B Renal vein thrombosis
4. C Vascular occlusion due to polycythaemia

An elderly patient has haematuria with back pain, polycythaemia and a painful varicocele. These features suggest a **left renal tumour** with increased production of erythropoietin and a possible occlusion of the left renal vein causing the varicocele. The raised Na, despite therapy with diuretics, suggests that the tumour is also producing renin (parathormone-related protein may also cause hypercalcaemia). An increasing number of renal cell carcinomas are now diagnosed incidentally on ultrasound. The main symptom is haematuria, the classical combination with low grade pyrexia and flank pain becoming more rare. These are very vascular tumours and, if inoperable, may successfully be embolised. The metastases (cannonball to the lung and lytic to the bone) are also very vascular and single chest metastases may be resected.

A normal brain scan excludes a haemorrhagic stroke, but not arterial occlusion. The affected side does not correspond to the carotid plaque.

Answers – Case History 2 (5 marks)

1. B Minimal change nephropathy
2. A Systemic steroids

The patient has nephrotic syndrome. Although the urinary protein loss is only marginally higher than microalbuminuria for an adult, in a child this would be equivalent to heavy proteinuria. IgA nephropathy is excluded by the absence of haematuria. Post-streptococcal immune complex nephritis usually presents within two to three weeks of an upper respiratory tract infection. Membranous and crescentic glomuleronephritis can be diagnosed on light microscopy. **Minimal change nephropathy** usually presents in early childhood but can be found in adults. The patients present with nephrotic syndrome but otherwise normal urine and are not usually hypertensive. Electron microscopy reveals fusion of the podocytes. Prognosis is good with oral steroids.

Answers – Case History 3 (8 marks)

1.

Best answers	a.	**Carpal tunnel syndrome**
	b.	**Secondary hyperparathyroidism**
Accepted answers	a.	Amyloid deposition
	b.	Hyperparathyroidism
Rejected answers	a.	Malignant bone tumour
	b.	Primary/Tertiary hyperparathyroidism/ Hypothyroidism

2.

Best answers	a.	**Nerve conduction studies**
	b.	**Parathormone levels**
Rejected answers	a.	US/CT scan of neck

3.

Best answers	a.	**Median nerve decompression**
	b.	**Calcium and vitamin D supplements**
Rejected answers	a.	Steroid injection
	b.	Parathyroidectomy

The patient has evidence of a sensory and motor neuropathy of the left median nerve. The most likely cause for this is **compression at the carpal tunnel** due to β2-microglobulin deposition in the flexor retinaculum. The fistula is not at a site where it can compress the median nerve and localised pressure effect from the brown tumour in the metacarpal would not cause a sensory deficit in the index finger. Treatment is by splitting of the flexor retinaculum.

In addition, the patient has radiological features of **hyperparathyroidism** with the hallmark sub-periosteal bone resorption. However, the calcium is on the low side indicating that this is secondary to inadequate replacement and has not yet become autonomous (tertiary hyperparathyroidism). The treatment at this stage is with a replacement to remove the stimulus of hypercalcaemia to the parathyroid glands.

Answers – Case History 4 (9 marks)

1.

Best answer: **Left sensory-neural impairment**
Accepted answer: Sensory-neural deafness
Rejected answers: Right sensory-neural deafness/Conduction defect

The sound transmitted through the skull vault on Weber's test is appreciated louder in the right ear. This either indicates nerve impairment of the left ear or relative reduction of the background noise transmitted through the right middle ear (middle ear conduction defect). However, as the relative relationship of air conduction > bone conduction is preserved in both ears, this indicates that both modalities are reduced on the left side giving an apparent normal result in Rinné's test.

2.
Best answer: **Lenticonus**
Accepted answer: Cataract/Lens abnormality
Rejected answer: Hypertensive retinopathy

3.
Best answer: **Alport's syndrome**
Accepted answer: Hereditary nephritis
Rejected answer: Vasculitis

4.
Best answer: **Progressive renal failure**
Rejected answer: Good prognosis with treatment

Alport's syndrome is a rare, inherited condition primarily affecting males. Inheritance is usually X-linked recessive although other traits have been described. The typical ocular abnormality is a conical deformity of the anterior aspect of the lens which may present as an apparent dark spot on fundoscopy. Sensory-neural nerve deafness is well described. The condition presents with haematuria and nephritis in childhood or adolescence. The renal failure is progressive.

Answers – Case History 5 (5 marks)

1. E IgA nephropathy
2. C Renal biopsy

IgA nephritis (Berger's disease) is a condition usually found in young, male adults. It frequently follows a non-specific upper respiratory tract infection without interval. There is mesangial deposition of IgA and C3 with evidence of focal proliferative glomerulonephritis on microscopy. HLA-DR4 is positive in 50%. It may present without obvious precipitating factor, prognosis is usually good but up to 10% develop chronic renal failure.

The main differential here is towards post-streptococcal GN, however there is typically an interval of two to three weeks between the upper respiratory tract infection and the main symptom is proteinuria, although haematuria can be seen. C3 is normal or high in IgA nephritis, but low in post-streptococcal GN. In addition, the history indicates that there was no response to the therapy with penicillin and macrolide antibiotics, making a viral infection more likely.

There is no history of purpura or arthralgia to suggest Henoch-Schönlein purpura.

Answers – Case History 6 (6 marks)

1. B Medullary sponge kidney

MSK is characterised by bilateral medullary nephrocalcinosis which is caused by formation of small stones in the dilated distal tubules.

2. A Wegener's granulomatosis
3. B Anti-neutrophilic cytoplasmic antibodies

The patient has a **pulmonary-renal syndrome**. The differential includes Goodpasture's syndrome, most vasculitides (in particular PAN, Wegener's and Churg-Strauss) and a primary pulmonary cause (i.e. pneumonia) with secondary renal impairment.

A combination of cavitating pulmonary nodules, a high ESR and crescentic (rapid progressive) glomerulonephritis is virtually diagnostic of **Wegener's granulomatosis**. The main differential is Goodpasture's syndrome with pulmonary haemorrhage (in which case, the CO-transfer factor would be increased). Pulmonary cavitation is not a feature and patients tend to be men under the age of 40.

In panarteritis nodosa, the lung changes seen on radiography are usually of pulmonary congestion and oedema, rarely due to focal infiltrates, although cavitation can be seen. P-ANCA is positive as opposed to C-ANCA in Wegener's. Angiography invariably shows small saccular aneurysms of small and medium-sized arteries in all affected organs.

Answers – Case History 7 (9 marks)

1.
Best answers: **Skeletal survey/Serum- and urine-electrophoresis**
Accepted answers: X-ray spine/Urine for Bence-Jones proteins/Serum globulin levels/β2 microglobulin levels/Steroid suppression test
Rejected answers: Bone marrow biopsy (invasive!)/Radio-isotope bone scan/Renal biopsy

2.
Best answer: **Multiple myeloma**
Accepted answer: Diffuse metastatic disease
Rejected answers: Paget's disease/Hyperparathyroidism

3.
Best answer: **Acute tubular necrosis**
Accepted answers: Acute renal failure/Exacerbation of myeloma kidney
Rejected answer: Renal obstruction

4.
Best answer: **Presence of light chains (Bence-Jones proteins)**
Accepted answer: Myeloma kidney
Rejected answer: Pre-existent renal failure

Two of the three following cardinal features have to be present for the diagnosis of **myeloma**:

1. Presence of monoclonal immunoglobulins in plasma/urine
2. Increase of plasma cells within bone marrow > 10% (normal < 8%)
3. Osteolytic (punched out) bone lesions

The presence of anaemia, hypercalcaemia and renal failure are poor prognostic factors in myeloma. Light chains (Kappa & Lambda) are present in up to 60% of IgG and IgA myeloma, and 100% in pure light chain myeloma. These are excreted in the urine and can obstruct the tubules. Administration of iv contrast is contraindicated! Bence-Jones proteins precipitate if urine is heated to 50 °C and dissolve again on further heating.

The well-defined bone lesions are caused by osteoclastic activity with virtually no sclerotic response unless a pathological factor occurs. The uptake of Technetium-labelled diphosphonates during a bone scan, however, is dependent on the activity of osteoblasts and false negative results are usually obtained.

Answers – Case History 8 (8 marks)

1. C Haemorrhage into cyst
2. A Adult polycystic disease
3. D *Pneumocystis carinii* pneumonia

The patient is of high risk for HIV infection. The combination of bilateral mid-zone infiltrates with or without cyst formation and desaturation on exercise are typically for PCP.

4. E Subarachnoid haemorrhage

For the purpose of the exam, history of adoption or foster parents should raise the suspicion about an inherited condition.

Adult polycystic disease is an autosomal dominant condition with a gene defect on the short arm of chromosome 16. Small cysts are formed in infancy which increase in size throughout life. Manifestation is usually in the second or third decade with renal failure, hypertension or clinical signs of haemorrhage into cyst (loin pain or haematuria). It can affect all parenchymatous organs; in particular, the liver, pancreas and spleen but huge cystic masses of both kidneys are the typical findings. The patients have an increased incidence of Berry aneurysms of the circle of Willis (in 20–25%) with the associated risk of subarachnoid haemorrhage.
A normal brain scan does **not** exclude SAH!

The autosomal recessive condition of infantile polycystic kidney disease is not a realistic differential as these present either antenatally or within the first five years of life. There is an associated risk of hepatic fibrosis and portal hypertension. Patients rarely reach the second decade. In both conditions, genetic counselling is essential. In APKD there is also a risk of hypertensive stroke which has to be differentiated from a subarachnoid haemorrhage. Other complications include renal calculi, UTI and rupture or infection of cyst.

NEPHROLOGY ANSWERS: DATA INTERPRETATIONS

Answers – Data Interpretation 1 (3 marks)

1. C Lactic acidosis Type A

The patient has a **raised anion gap** $[Na^+ + K^+] - [Cl^- + HCO_3^-] = 29$ mmol/l. Normal range 10–18 mmol/l. In the context given, this is most likely to be due to shock and tissue hypoxia indicating Type A, rather than a toxic cause, such as biguanide therapy or salicylate overdose.

For the purpose of the exam, if the chloride is given (particularly if double figures only), this should immediately prompt for a calculation of the anion gap.

Answers – Data Interpretation 2 (4 marks)

1. E Haemolytic uraemic syndrome
2. C *E. coli* infection

HUS is a childhood syndrome characterised by intravascular haemolysis (micro-angiopathic haemolysis), thrombocytopaenia and acute renal failure. Precipitating causes are respiratory tract infections and gastro-enteritis with *E. coli* O 157. The prognosis is usually very good.

Aplastic crises in children with congenital haemogloblinopathies (i.e. sickle-cell) occur after infection with Parvovirus B19 (5th disease, slapped cheek disease).

Answers – Data Interpretation 3 (2 marks)

1. B Combined respiratory and metabolic acidosis

The patient is clearly acidotic. O_2 tension is decreased, CO_2 tension is increased indicating respiratory failure in keeping with chronic COAD. However, there is no compensatory increase of the bicarbonate which is reduced below normal levels indicating an associated metabolic acidosis. The oxygen saturation of > 80% indicates an arterial sample. Conversion from kiloPascal to millimetres Hg is done by multiplying by an approximate factor of 7.5 (10 kPa = 75 mmHg).

Answers – Data Interpretation 4 (4 marks)

1.
Best answer: **Renal tubular acidosis Type I**
Accepted answer: Renal tubular acidosis
Rejected answer: Diuretic therapy

2.
Best answers: **Primary biliary cirrhosis/Chronic active hepatitis**
Accepted answer: Vitamin D intoxication
Rejected answer: Hypergammaglobulinaemia

The patient has a hypokalaemic acidosis, this constellation is highly suggestive of **renal tubular acidosis**. The age and the presence of renal calculi suggests RTA Type I (distal tubular acidification defect). This may be inherited by any of the traits or may be secondary to a variety of diseases. Hypergammaglobulinaema is excluded by the normal globulin factions.

Answers – Data Interpretation 5 (4 marks)

1. B Urate stones
2. D Bicarbonate supplements

Uric acid stones are not uncommon in patients with ileostomies. The increased loss of fluid and bicarbonate through the stoma results in the production of concentrated acidic urine, which causes precipitation of uric acid. Alkalinization of urine will prevent stone formation.

Urate and **X**anthine stones are radiol**ux**ent.

Answers – Data Interpretation 6 (3 marks)

1. A Wilms' tumour

Nephroblastoma is a malignant childhood tumour of the kidney, with the main differential being a neuroblastoma of the sympathetic chain (frequently arising in the adrenal gland). Infection as a complication of horseshoe kidney or VU reflux is excluded by the absence of protein and white cells in the urine.

Answers – Data Interpretation 7 (4 marks)

1. A Aplastic anaemia
2. D Drug-induced glomerulonephritis

The patient has a pancytopaenia and heavy proteinuria. The renal biopsy is consistent with the **membranous glomerulonephritis**. Both features can either be due to therapy with gold or penicillamine. Methotrexate, as a folate antagonist, can cause macrocytic anaemia.

Answers – Data Interpretation 8 (4 marks)

1.
Best answer: **Rhabdomyolysis**
Rejected answer: Acute renal failure

2.
Best answer: **Electric shock**
Accepted answers: Epileptic fit/Alcohol excess/Hypothermia

There is a marked discrepancy between the increase of creatinine and urea as well as the liver specific ALT and the AST which is also contained within striated muscle. The extensive tissue damage from electrocution causes hyperkalaemia, calcium levels may be low.

Answers – Data Interpretation 9 (4 marks)

1. D Lesch-Nyhan syndrome
2. B X-linked recessive enzyme defect

Lesch-Nyhan syndrome is characterised by a reduction (< 1%) in activity of hypoxanthin-guanin-phosphoribosil transferase which leads to a chronic increase in uric acid, with all the symptoms of hyperuricaemia and progressive renal failure. This is associated with a variety of neurological symptoms, classically with a tendency to self mutilation. The patient is too young for 'simple' gout. Gout arthropathy causes well-defined (punched out) deep erosions along the shaft of the phalanges, adjacent to, but not necessarily involving the articular surface. Involvement is usually unilateral but can be bilateral but asymmetrical. Calcified tophi indicate a chronic form.

Answers – Data Interpretation 10 (6 marks)

1.
Best answer: **Bilateral renal vein thrombosis**
Accepted answer: Renal vein thrombosis
Rejected answers: Acute on chronic renal failure/Acute exacerbation of lupus

2.
Best answers: **Anticoagulation/Warfarin**
Accepted answers: Heparin/Dialysis
Rejected answers: High dose steroids/Immunosuppressants

3.
Best answers: **Poor prognosis/Renal function unlikely to recover**
Accepted answer: Chronic renal failure
Rejected answer: Good prognosis with treatment

Thrombotic episodes are common in **nephrotic syndrome**, in particular in the context of membranous glomerulonephritis. In membranous nephropathy, up to 30% undergo spontaneous remission, but progression to end-stage renal failure occurs in the majority of patients.

Thrombosis classically affects the renal veins, urinary loss of anti-thrombin III has been implicated. If there is venous infarction of the kidney, this is associated with loin pain, as well as haematuria and increased proteinuria. If adequate collateral circulation is present, the event may be subclinical. Rapid deterioration of renal function indicates bilateral venous occlusion.

If the patients are at very high risk of pulmonary embolism and require anticoagulation, heparin may be ineffective, as anti-thrombin III is usually low. Warfarin, as is it largely protein-bound, has to be administered with great care.

Answers – Data Interpretation 11 (5 marks)

1. C Renal artery stenosis
2. D Renal artery angioplasty

The patient has a raised baseline aldosterone and renin. The aldosterone drops to normal values after captopril, indicating a **secondary hyperaldosteronism**. In Conn's syndrome, the aldosterone levels are not affected.

An increase in renin concentration by up to 50% can be seen in essential hypertension and this is non-specific. However, an increment of more than 100% is highly suggestive of renal artery stenosis.

Answers – Data Interpretation 12 (5 marks)

1. C Salt-wasting nephropathy
2. E Renal tuberculosis

The patient clearly has **salt wastage** which is an unspecific indicator of tubular damage. Causes include analgesics, chronic infection (including TB!), and obstruction, heavy metals (including Wilson's disease), amyloid, recovering ATN and nephrocalcinosis.

Sterile pyuria (> 10 white cells/μl) is strongly suggestive of **TB**, but may also be seen in Stone disease, interstitial nephritis and papillary necrosis.

Answers – Data Interpretation 13 (4 marks)

1. D Cervical swab
2. A Gonorrhoea

In a small proportion of men and up to 30% of women, **gonorrhoea** can remain asymptomatic. Complications include ascending salpingitis and pelvic inflammatory disease, prostatitis, reactive arthritis (especially monarthritis of knee), septicaemia, endocarditis, and perihepatitis (Fitz-Hugh-Curtis syndrome). The Gram-negative diplococci require special media for culture, but can be identified on Gram stains. A co-existent venereal disease, i.e. syphilis, has to be considered.

Answers – Data Interpretation 14 (4 marks)

1. E Urine cytology and radio-isotope bone scan
2. A Transitional cell carcinoma

Occupational diseases of the chemical worker are **transitional cell carcinoma** due to aniline dyes and haemangiosarcoma of the liver due to PVC poisoning (this also causes resorption of the mid portions of the terminal phalanges in the hands). TCC presents with haematuria and features of renal obstruction. They are best demonstrated by cystoscopy and retrograde pyelography. However, urine cytology and an IVU for demonstrating the level of obstruction should be performed first, and this patient also has evidence of metastatic bone disease.

Answers – Data Interpretation 15 (5 marks)

1. B Allergic interstitial nephritis
2. E Withdrawal of all medication

The symptoms described are of osteoarthritis and not of an inflammatory arthropathy. Her GP would have treated her with simple analgesics or non-steroidal anti-inflammatory drugs (NSAIDs). One month later, she has heavy proteinuria as well as glycosuria indicating both glomerular and tubular damage.

NSAIDs are a common cause of **allergic interstitial nephritis** as are antibiotics. Other features may include fever, arthralgia, eosinophilia, haematuria and acute renal failure. The diagnosis can be confirmed by renal biopsy showing interstitial lymphocytic infiltrates. Withdrawal of the offending drug will usually lead to spontaneous resolution, in severe cases steroids may be required.

Answers – Data Interpretation 16 (4 marks)

1. D *Treponema pallidum* haemagglutination test
2. B Jarisch-Herxheimer reaction

For the purpose of the exam, a travelling salesman and the Far East equal an infectious, usually venereal disease. The clinical features are of **secondary syphilis** which can produce aseptic meningitis. The 'snail track ulcers' are infective, but microscopy and culture are unreliable. TPHA is a useful screening test, FTA (fluorescence-treponema-antibody-absorption test) is more specific and confirms active infection. VDRL test is non-specific but a reasonable monitor of disease activity.

Jarisch-Herxheimer reaction is caused by release of large amounts of endotoxins due to good response to antibiotics. It usually occurs within 24 hours and can be ameliorated by prednisolone cover.

Treatment of syphilis is with parenteral (1.2 g/im) depot penicillin for two weeks.

NEUROLOGY ANSWERS: CASE HISTORIES

Answers – Case History 1 (7 marks)

1. C Carotid Doppler
2. E Chronic subdural haematoma
3. A Neurosurgical referral

An anticoagulated elderly patient has a mixture of neurological symptoms of subacute onset. The intermittent and fluctuating nature points towards a space-occupying lesion rather than an ischaemic process. A left-sided carotid problem would also localise to the other side. The most likely diagnosis is **subdural haematoma**. These may occur spontaneously without a history of trauma or anticoagulation. The two most important investigations are a prothrombin time/INR and a CT brain scan.

On a CT scan with brain settings, freshly clotted blood appears white. This turns to the same 'greyness' (isodense) as brain substance after two-three weeks and appears as dark as water (CSF in ventricles) after approximately one month. The sequence is dependent on haemoglobin concentration, clotting factors, including warfarin, and recurrent haemorrhage.

Clinical symptoms may be insidious with confusion, ataxia or incontinence. If symptomatic, neurosurgical decompression should be considered.

Hyponatraemia should alert to the possibility of inappropriate ADH-secretion which may be caused by essentially any pathology within the head (tumour, haemorrhage, raised intracranial pressure, infection); any pathology within the chest (tumour, infection, particularly Legionella, empyema), drugs, acute porphyria and lymphoma.

Answers – Case History 2 (8 marks)

1. A Chest X-ray
2. C von Hippel-Lindau syndrome
3. D Bilateral renal cell carcinomata
4. C 40–50%

von Hippel-Lindau syndrome (retino-cerebellar haemangioblastosis) is characterised by haemangioblastoma formation in the eye, the cerebellum and, less commonly, in other organs. Cysts are frequently found in liver, spleen and kidneys. Large, benign angio-myolipoma can be found in the kidneys, but the combination of hypertension and haematuria is very suggestive of the commonly found (up to 40%!) renal cell carcinoma. The tumours are frequently multicentric and commonly bilateral.

Although staging with a CT abdomen will be required, exclusion of metastases with a chest X-ray is more important in the first instance.

Polycythaemia is found in a significant minority, erythropoietin is produced by the hypernephroma as well as the cerebellar haemangio-blastoma.

The defect is localised in chromosome 3, transmission is autosomal dominant with 80–90% penetrance, hence the patient has a 1:2 chance of acquiring the defect with a very high likelihood of this being expressed.

Answers – Case History 3 (7 marks)

1. B Guillain-Barré syndrome
2. C Pulmonary function tests
3. B Ventilation

The patient has a distal neuropathy which is also involving both facial nerves. This is associated with a sensory neuropathy affecting the spino-thalamic tracts as well as the dorsal columns (soft touch).

This is of fairly acute onset, the CSF shows a characteristically high protein with normal microscopy. This can cause communicating hydrocephalus due to impaired re-absorption of CSF.

The reduction in nerve conduction is typical for a demyelinating polyneuritis.

Treatment of **GBS** is mainly supportive, respiratory depression may require ventilation.

Tetanus and botulism affect the motor endplates only (as does myasthenia gravis), herpes encephalitis may cause UMN-signs but not a peripheral neuropathy.

Answers – Case History 4 (7 marks)

1.
Best answer: **Duchenne muscular dystrophy**
Accepted answer: Becker's muscular dystrophy
Rejected answers: Guillain-Barré syndrome/Myositis poliomyelitis

2.
Best answer: **Creatinine phosphokinase levels**
Accepted answers: Muscle biopsy/Genetic screening
Rejected answer: Virology screen

3.
Best answer: **Death before 20**
Accepted answer: Very poor
Rejected answer: Death in middle-age

DMD is an X-linked recessive disorder with some spontaneous mutations and an incidence of 1:3,000. The boys manifest the disease within five years, become disabled within 10 years and die before 20 years of age. Clinically, there is a progressive proximal myopathy, the boys become unwilling to run and play and they need to 'climb up their legs' to an erect position (Gower's sign).

An associated cardiomyopathy is frequently found, CPK levels are raised hundred to two-hundred-fold and EMG show evidence of myopathy. Muscle biopsy (second-line test in a 4-year-old) shows necrosis with regeneration, disorganisation and fatty replacement.

The main differential is with Becker's dystrophy which manifests in later childhood (< 10), leads to disability in the 20's and death occurs in middle-age. Cardiac involvement is unusual, inheritance is also X-linked recessive.

Answers – Case History 5 (7 marks)

1. B Blood film
2. A Subacute combined degeneration of the cord
3. C Folate replacement

SACD is a consequence of protracted vitamin B_{12} deficiency, usually caused by pernicious anaemia. Classically there is evidence of upper motor neurone as well as lower motor neurone defects in the legs, as well as a mixed sensory deficit with emphasis on the posterior columns (hence 'combined' degeneration). The longest nerves are affected earliest in a peripheral neuropathy and the arc of the spinal reflex is lost distally in the ankle while upper motor neurone signs still dominate more proximally (plantar reflexes are not a spinal reflex).

There is no evidence of liver damage to suggest alcohol abuse as the underlying cause. The pancytopenia supports a diagnosis of pernicious anaemia. A blood film would show macrocytosis and hypersegmented neutrophils.

As B_{12} and folate deficiency often co-exists the replacement with folate may acutely exacerbate the B_{12} deficiency as the blood cells begin to regenerate. The peripheral neuropathy usually responds well to B_{12} replacement, whereas cord and brain damage may persist.

Reduction in amplitude of the motor neurone potentials with preserved conduction velocity indicate an axonal disease process.

Answers – Case History 6 (8 marks)

1. E Paraneoplastic syndrome
2. D Response to exercise
3. C Ectopic ACTH secretion
4. A Chest X-ray

A complex picture, however the neurological problem can be classified as a lower motor neurone deficit affecting the peripheral system symmetrically, but also involving the cranial nerves. Being better in the evening suggests improvement with exercise which is strongly suggestive of **Eaton-Lambert syndrome**, a myasthenic-myopathic syndrome which is a paraneoplastic manifestation of small cell carcinoma of the bronchus. It is characterised by a defect in release of acetyl choline and as an important differential to myasthenia gravis it improves with repetition. In addition, the patient has evidence of ectopic ACTH-secretion with diabetes, high sodium, low potassium and truncal obesity. A Cushingoid state may also cause a proximal myopathy, however this does not improve with exercise.

Ectopic PTH-secretion (or PTH-related hormone) is usually found with *squamous cell carcinoma.*

Hypertrophic pulmonary osteo-arthropathy (HPOA) is normally found with squamous and adeno-carcinoma.

Small cell carcinoma is aggressive and spreads quickly even with a small primary tumour, but is the one that responds well to chemotherapy.

Answers – Case History 7 (9 marks)

1. A Botulism
2. B Arterial blood gases
3. E Anti-toxin
4. D Admit to intensive care and inform Public Health

The acute onset of a global neurological syndrome characterised by paralysis is suggestive of an acute infection or toxic effects. The absence of focal symptoms and normal blood parameters essentially exclude a cerebral abscess. Tetanus is characterised by tonic seizures in a conscious patient; rabies has a protracted onset with features of encephalitis.

Organophosphate poisoning is characterised by strong cholinergic/ muscarinic effects and not by a flaccid paralysis.

Spores of ***Clostridium botulinum*** are found in soil. Under anaerobic conditions (home canned meat, pickled vegetables, home-made wine) the most potent toxin known to man is produced. It is destroyed by heat, the earliest manifestations, besides diarrhoea and vomiting, are diplopia. The eye muscles, in particular lateral rectus, are the best innervated muscles in the body and most sensitive to toxic effects. Treatment is with anti-toxins and supportive measures, if the patient survives the respiratory paralysis, outcome is usually good.

Answers – Case History 8 (9 marks)

1. E Left-sided thoracic tumour
2. C Superior orbital fissure meningioma
3. A Right sensory-neural deficit
4. D Neurofibromatosis Type II

The patient has features of **Brown-Séquard syndrome**. A unilateral lesion causes an ipsilateral upper motor neurone deficit and ipsilateral posterior column signs. As the spino-thalamic fibres cross in the spine at segmental level, deficits to sharp pain and temperature are found on the contra-lateral side below the level of the lesion. Hyperaesthesia at the costal margin indicates a lesion in the mid-thoracic spine. A disc problem would not cause posterior column signs.

The motor deficit in the left eye affects the 3rd as well as the 6th cranial nerve, the lack of parasympathetic drive indicates compression. The 3rd, 4th and 6th cranial nerves run together in the lateral wall of the cavernous sinus and enter the orbit in the superior orbital fissure. Cavernous sinus thrombosis is a dramatic event with chemosis and proptosis of the affected side.

In **Weber's test**, the tuning fork placed centrally on the forehead is appreciated louder in an ear with conduction deficit (the background noise from the environment is reduced and the sound conducted through the skull to the functioning nerve is appreciated louder). In a sensory-neural problem the sound is conducted less well through the damaged nerve and, therefore, lateralisation is to the normal side.

In **Rinné's test**, a middle ear problem causing a conduction deficit will lead to bone conduction through the mastoid being appreciated louder than air conduction. With a neural deficit, both modalities are reduced equally, air conduction still being appreciated better.

The patient has multiple defects at different sites caused by nerve compression, the most likely cause is multiple benign tumours as seen in Type II (central) neurofibromatosis. Bilateral acoustic neuromas are the classical presentation, it is transmitted autosomal dominant on chromosome 22. The patients rarely have skin manifestations and there is no association with phaeochromocytoma/MEN or the other typical features of NF1 (autosomal dominant chromosome 17). The two are separate entities, NF1 is 9 times more common.

NEUROLOGY ANSWERS: DATA INTERPRETATIONS

Answers – Data Interpretation 1 (4 marks)

1. D Tuberculous meningitis
2. D Communicating hydrocephalus

The combination of mild CSF lymphocytosis, increased protein and reduced glucose suggests **TB meningitis**. This affects the basal aspects of the brain and may involve cranial nerves at this site. The high protein reduces CSF re-absorption and causes communicating hydrocephalus (communicating as no CSF spaces are obstructed). This may cause brain stem descent with false localising signs.

Cysticercosis causes focal mass lesions causing seizures or focal signs.

Answers – Data Interpretation 2 (4 marks)

1. E Drug screen
2. B Periodic paralysis

An acute presentation of a generalised lower motor neurone syndrome involving the bulb. The patient is not dehydrated to suggest a 'rave' party, myasthenic crisis cannot be excluded but is unlikely, McArdle's syndrome (myophosphorylase deficiency) causes fatiguability but myoglobin is found in the urine which tests falsely positive for blood on dipstix.

The striking hypokalaemia in a young patient should alert to **hypokalaemic periodic paralysis**, an autosomal dominant trait presenting in childhood with remission in the third decade. Attacks last several hours, are usually self-limiting but respond to administration of potassium.

A hyperkalaemic form has also been described.

Answers – Data Interpretation 3 (5 marks)

1. B Cerebral sarcoid
2. A Chest X-ray

The patient has a lower motor neurone palsy of the facial nerve associated with CSF lymphocytosis and mildly raised protein. The features are consistent with **cerebral sarcoidosis**. The facial nerves are directly affected, both sides can be involved simultaneously. Involvement of the parotid glands may indicate Heerfordt syndrome (uveo-parotid fever). Ophthalmology referral for assessment of uveitis should be considered. A benign pleomorphic adenoma of the parotid does not cause CSF changes.

Answers – Data Interpretation 4 (6 marks)

1. C Subarachnoid haemorrhage
2. D Adult polycystic kidney disease
3. B Ultrasound abdomen

The xanthochromia indicates that blood was present in the subarachnoid space prior to the traumatic lumbar puncture. Xanthochromia (yellow staining) of CSF occurs 2–4 hrs after haemorrhage. A normal brain CT does not exclude a SAH.

The usual cause for this is a ruptured Berry aneurysm, these are associated with adult polycystic kidney disease as indicated by the renal failure and the flank mass. IV contrast *does not improve* visualisation of subarachnoid blood.

The capillary angiomata found in Sturge-Weber syndrome on the leptomeninges cause seizures and focal cerebral atrophy, but tend not to bleed.

Answers – Data Interpretation 5 (5 marks)

1. E Acute intermittent porphyria
2. D Chlorpromazine

Acute psychosis, abdominal pain, peripheral polyneuropathy and hyponatraemia represent the full house of acute intermittent porphyria. Variegated porphyria has identical features plus photosensitivity.

The BNF contains a list of drugs unsafe in porphyria.

Answers – Data Interpretation 6 (6 marks)

1.

Best answer: **Pneumococcal meningitis**
Accepted answer: Bacterial meningitis
Rejected answers: Meningitis/Meningococcal meningitis

2.
Best answer: **Intravenous cefotaxime**
Accepted answer: Intravenous penicillin
Rejected answer: Antibiotics

3.
Best answers: **Pneumococcal vaccination/Notification of Public Health**
Accepted answers: Antibiotic prophylaxis to contacts/Antibiotic prophylaxis for patient
Rejected answers: Barrier nursing/Nasal swab

Asplenia in sickle cell disease or after splenectomy requires pneumococcal vaccination. In children additional anaphylactic prophylaxis is recommended. Clinically, the main differential is meningococcal meningitis, although these are Gram-negative diplococci. Treatment of choice is currently cefotaxime (March 2000). Meningitis is a notifiable disease.

Answers – Data Interpretation 7 (6 marks)

1. D Impaired glucose tolerance
2. B Hypergonadotropic hypogonadism
3. A Myotonic dystrophy

The combination of diffuse lower motor neurone lesion, cardiac conduction defects and a visual problem not corrected by glasses (cataract!) should alert to **myotonic dystrophy**.

An autosomal dominant condition associated with impaired glucose tolerance, primary hypogonadism and impaired intellectual function.

The patient is too old for Friedreich's ataxia; Kallmann's syndrome is characterised by reduced gonadotrophins and anosmia, but no neuromuscular problems.

Answers – Data Interpretation 8 (3 marks)

1. A CT scan of brain
2. E Benign intracranial hypertension

The young woman is overweight and on the pill. Two risk factors for benign intracranial hypertension, which is confirmed by lumbar puncture. The ventricular system is most likely to show normal appearances on CT scan. The importance of the CT scan is to exclude an obstructing lesion and this should be done prior to LP. Treatment is required to prevent blindness. If weight reduction and stopping the pill fails, repeated lumbar punctures or a shunt may be required. The condition may be primary or secondary.

Answers – Data Interpretation 9 (5 marks)

1. C Thyroid function tests
2. E Hypothyroidism and pernicious anaemia

The patient has extensive features of profound hypothyroidism with acute confusion/delusion (**myxoedema madness**). Alcohol abuse is the most likely differential, but the normal liver function tests are strongly against this.

Hypothyroidism is associated with pernicious anaemia, but may cause a macrocytic anaemia on its own, although normochromic normocytic is more common.

Hyperlipidaemia may result in spurious hyponatraemia.

Answers – Data Interpretation 10 (6 marks)

1. D Listeriosis
2. A Blood cultures
3. B iv erythromycin

Listeria monocytogenes is a ubiquitous facultatively anaerobic bacillus which is heat resistant to 60 °C (unpasteurised milk!). It becomes invasive in immune-suppressed patients and pregnancy where it causes meningitis, septicaemia and abortion. It is classically transmitted in blue cheeses but can be found in most poorly prepared foodstuffs.
Treatment is either with a combination of broad spectrum penicillin and gentamycin, alternatively erythromycin or 4-quinolones.
Viral infection and SLE would cause lymphocytosis.

Answers – Data Interpretation 11 (4 marks)

1. D Hereditary sensory-motor neuropathy
2. A Normal fundi

The patient has a neuropathy affecting sensor and motor systems. There is no evidence of upper motor neurone signs, making SACD and neurone-syphilis unlikely. Friedreich's ataxia is unlikely due to the absence of cerebellar signs, also involvement of the lateral spino-thalamic tracts is not usually seen.

Answers – Data Interpretation 12 (6 marks)

1. E Wernicke's syndrome
2. C iv thiamine
3. B Oral chlordiazepoxide

The macrocytic anaemia and chronic subdural haemorrhage in a vagrant suggest chronic alcohol abuse. The rapid onset of the typical triad of ataxia, confusion and nystagmus are diagnostic of **Wernicke's encephalopathy**. The chronic thiamine deficiency is acutely exacerbated by the high carbohydrate intake with hospital food. This results in haemorrhagic necrosis in the limbic system, particularly the mamillary bodies and the brain stem. IV thiamine or combined vitamin B compounds need to be given with great care due to possible anaphylaxis.

The impaired clotting due to liver damage forbids intramuscular injections. Administration of hypertonic saline can result in central pontine myelinolysis.

Answers – Data Interpretation 13 (4 marks)

1. B Syringobulbia
2. D MR scan of cervical spine

The patient has low motor neurone signs in the upper limbs and upper motor neurone signs in the lower limbs, indicating a lesion in the cervical cord. In addition, there is dissociate sensory loss (light touch is predominantly conducted in the posterior columns), typical features of a syrinx. However, the lower motor neurone lesion of the 12th cranial nerve indicates that it extends up into the brain stem in keeping with **syringobulbia**.

Answers – Data Interpretation 14 (5 marks)

1. B Right optic atrophy
2. E Multiple sclerosis

The patient has a **right afferent pupillary defect**. This indicates damage to the right optic nerve as the light shone in the right eye does not cause ipsilateral or contralateral pupillary constriction.

Associated with walking difficulties in a young woman it is most likely due to **demyelination**.

Neurosyphilis causes a small irregular pupil that constricts on convergence but not to light (Argyll-Robertson pupil).

The pale retinal tumours of tuberose sclerosis can also cause blindness. Other features are epilepsy, low intelligence, adenoma sebaceum (hence the acronym EpiLoIA) and the other rashes, ash leaf macule and Shagreen patch.

A Holmes-Adie pupil is a large pupil with sluggish reaction to light and accommodation, it is of no clinical significance other than it is associated with reduced tendon reflexes in young women.

RESPIRATORY MEDICINE ANSWERS: CASE HISTORIES

Answers – Case History 1 (9 marks)

1. D Compensated respiratory alkalosis
2. C High-resolution CT scan
3. E Asbestosis
4. C Pleural encasement

The wife of a plumber 'contracting' **asbestos-related lung disease** is an old classic of the exam. This is a well-documented occurrence from washing the husband's clothes (!).

The initial lung function tests show a restrictive defect with hyperventilation and mild compensatory reduction in bicarbonate. In combination with the clinical findings this indicates *asbestosis* (= asbestos induced pulmonary fibrosis). Investigation of choice is a thin section CT.

The spectrum of asbestos-related lung disease includes calcified pleural plaques, pleural thickening/encasement, recurrent *benign* pleural effusions, adeno-carcinoma (particularly in smokers) and pleural/ peritoneal mesothelioma.

The latency of complications is 10–30 years and the expected peak incidence of asbestosis and mesothelioma is around 2010!

The subsequent deterioration of the lung function with exaggeration of the restrictive defect in the presence of a relatively normal transfer coefficient indicate an extra-pulmonary restriction.

Answers – Case History 2 (9 marks)

1.
Best answer: **Pneumocystis carinii pneumonia**
Accepted answer: Pressure change during long-haul flight
Rejected answers: Pulmonary embolism/Pneumonia

2.
Best answers: **HIV-infection/AIDS**
Accepted answers: Immune-suppression/Lymphoma/Viral/atypical pneumonia
Rejected answers: Marfan's disease/Legionnaire's disease

3.

Best answers: **Blood film/differential/Sputum microscopy and culture/High-resolution CT/AIDS test after counselling**
Accepted answers: Transbronchial lung biopsy/Repeat blood gases after exercise/Blood cultures/Social history
Rejected answers: AIDS test/CD4-count

4.

Best answer: **High-dose co-trimoxazole**
Accepted answers: Co-trimoxazole/Pentamidine/Trimetrexate
Rejected answers: Aspiration of pneumothorax/Chest drain

A small pneumothorax of this size in a young male should not cause respiratory compromise to this degree. In addition, the patient has features of infection as well as immune-compromise (pancytopenia). The social history strongly points toward **PC-pneumonia in HIV infection**. AIDS testing must not be performed without counselling, sneaky ways of establishing CD4 counts are unethical.

Other differentials of chest infection, i.e. atypical Mycobacterium, other fungi and CMV also need to be considered.

PCP typically presents with bilateral hazy mid-zone shadowing, the chest X-ray may however be normal and a pneumothorax is present in up to 10%. It is a marker disease for HIV. Proof is by silver staining of sputum or lung biopsy.

Answers – Case History 3 (6 marks)

1. A Wegener's granulomatosis
2. C Lateral chest X-ray
3. B iv cyclophosphamide

The patient has a systemic disease affecting eyes, chest and kidneys. In addition, 9% of the differential is unaccounted for which is likely to represent eosinophils. Of the vasculitides, pulmonary nodules are typical for **Wegener's granulomatosis**. These frequently cavitate.

Renal biopsy and estimation of c-ANCA is required. In view of the occupation extrinsic allergic alveolitis has to be excluded. Lateral chest X-ray will not provide any further information. The nasal passage and the sinuses are usually involved and diagnosis can also be made on biopsy from this site. Eye involvement and retro-bulbar granulomata are common.

Treatment is with cyclophosphamide and additional steroids if required.

Answers – Case History 4 (7 marks)

1.
Best answers: **Transbronchial lung biopsy/High-resolution CT scan/24-hour ECG monitoring/Auto-antibody screen/Arterial blood gases**
Accepted answers: Radioisotope gallium scan/Steroid suppression test/ Sputum microscopy and culture/Lymph node biopsy
Rejected answers: Serum ACE levels/Kveim test

2.
Best answer: **Sarcoidosis with cardiac involvement**
Accepted answers: Sarcoidosis/Lymphoma/SLE
Rejected answers: Vitamin D intoxication/Rheumatoid arthritis

3.
Best answers: **High-dose steroids/Cardiac pacing**
Accepted answers: Forced diuresis/Chloroquine/Immune suppressants, Cardiology referral
Rejected answers: Anti-tuberculous therapy/Cardiac transplant

A young Afro-Caribbean woman presents with a systemic disease characterised by a restrictive pulmonary defect, lymphadenopathy, polyarthralgia and cardiac conduction defect. In the presence of hypercalcaemia, the diagnosis is **sarcoidosis**.

The ECG findings indicate a bi-fascicular block (RBBB plus left-anterior hemi-block) with an associated first degree AV-block. This heralds a tri-fascicular block/complete AV block and pacing must be considered. Acute sarcoidosis responds well to steroids. Chronic pulmonary sarcoid and cardiac involvement have a poor prognosis.

Answers – Case History 5 (8 marks)

1. D Aspergilloma
2. C CT scan
3. A Emphysema
4. D Surgery

Aspergillus fumigatus is a fungus which causes three distinct clinical pictures:

- Allergic bronchial pulmonary aspergillosis (ABPA) – a hypersensitivity reaction typically occurring in young male patients presenting with asthma. Mucoid plugs are expectorated and the patient develops *proximal* bronchiectasis.
- Invasive aspergillosis – in immune-compromised patients, the fungus can become invasive and causes cavitating pneumonia, usually in the apices.
- Aspergilloma – a fungus ball develops in a pre-existing cavity, usually following TB. It can remain asymptomatic for a long time, but haemoptysis is the usual complication. Surgical excision is the treatment of choice, direct intra-cavity injection of antibiotics is a second-line treatment option.

Answers – Case History 6 (7 marks)

1. E Chest X-ray
2. D Kartagener's syndrome
3. A 0%

Kartagener's syndrome (Max Kartagener, 1933, Swiss physician) or immotile ciliae syndrome is characterised by the recurrent upper (sinusitis) and lower respiratory tract infections leading to bronchiectasis. The defect in ciliary motility affects the bronchial escalator as well as the motility of sperm and the male patients are *infertile*. It is associated with dextrocardia/complete situs inversus as indicated by the ECG findings.

Answers – Case History 7 (7 marks)

1. B Serum phosphate
2. A Squamous cell carcinoma of the lung
3. E Forced diuresis and chest X-ray

Hyperparathyroidism occurs as a paraneoplastic manifestation of **squamous cell carcinoma of the lung**. This is due to secretion of parathormone-related peptide (PTH-rp), its effect is confirmed by a low phosphate. Bone metastases and Paget's disease are essentially excluded by the normal bone scan, multiple myeloma is extremely unlikely in the presence of normal (< 8%) plasma cell count in the bone marrow. The hypercalcaemia of ectopic PTH secretion does not suppress as well in the *steroid suppression test* as sarcoidosis, myeloma, Addison's disease or hypervitaminosis D. Treatment in the first instance is with aggressive rehydration and added diuretics. Removal of the primary tumour usually results in a dramatic drop of the serum calcium within 48 hours.

Answers – Case History 8 (7 marks)

1. D Sarcoidosis
2. E Skull X-ray and urine osmolality
3. C Central diabetes insipidus

Eosinophilic granuloma is the benign end of the spectrum of *Langerhans cell histiocytosis* (formerly histiocytosis X), e.g. usually presents in early adulthood with respiratory problems, most of the patients are smokers. The typical findings are reticulo-nodular changes which, if progress, result in cyst formation and honeycombing. The cysts may rupture and pneumothorax is common. The lung volumes are usually preserved. It may affect other parts of the body, notably the bones where the commonest site is the parietal bone in the skull. The classical appearance is of punched out lesions with a bevelled edge. Involvement of the pituitary may cause central diabetes insipidus. (The patient has a serum osmolality of 305 mosmol/kg and polyuria). The disease is often self-limiting, treatment with steroids is sometimes effective. Aggressive forms of childhood (Hand-Schüller-Christian disease) and the progressive form of infancy (Abt-Letterer-Siwe disease) carry a poor prognosis, and are associated with more systemic features, such as skin involvement, lymphadenopathy and hepatosplenomegaly.

Tuberose sclerosis and neurofibromatosis may also lead to cystic changes in the lungs.

Lymphangio-leiomyomatosis is a progressive hyperplasia of smooth muscles in the lymphatics, leading to lymphatic obstruction. This is also associated with lung cysts, it is virtually limited to women and the prognosis is poor unless pulmonary transplantation is performed. Lung cysts and pneumothoraces are not a feature of sarcoidosis.

Answers – Case History 9 (5 marks)

1. A Acute epiglottitis
2. A Urgent ENT referral and intubation

Acute infective epiglottitis is a respiratory emergency caused by infection with *Haemophilus influenzae*. This may lead to acute upper airway obstruction, although this is much rarer in adults than in children. Instrumentation of the mouth should only be performed by experts as this may provoke airway closure. Treatment is with iv antibiotics (amoxicillin resistance is now common), humidification of room air and early intubation/tracheostomy to safeguard the airways.

Laryngitis (croup) is caused by viral infection, the commonest is para-influenza virus.

Answers – Case History 10 (6 marks)

1. B Auto-antibody screen
2. E Cryptogenic fibrosing alveolitis
3. A Auto-immune chronic active hepatitis

The patient has a severe, restrictive lung defect with radiographic evidence of active alveolitis (ground-glass). **Cryptogenic fibrosing alveolitis** usually presents insidiously in middle-aged men, although a rare fulminant form has been described (Hamman-Rich syndrome). It is associated with other auto-immune conditions, such as CAH, coeliac disease and inflammatory bowel disease. Diagnosis can usually be made on a combination of the clinical findings and thin-section CT, although broncho-alveolar lavage or lung biopsy may be required.

Chronic active hepatitis (CAH) is characterised by a hepatic increase in transaminases and markedly raised immunoglobulins. Liver biopsy gives the diagnosis.

Answers – Case History 11 (6 marks)

1. A Chronic myeloid leukaemia in blast crisis
2. C Cytomegaly virus
3. B Isolation and sputum examination

The patient has **CML in blast transformation**. She is susceptible to atypical and fungal infections. Besides TB and MAI, invasive

aspergillosis has to be considered as a further cavitating pneumonia.
Staphylococcus and Klebsiella are bacterial causes of cavitating pneumonia.
PCP, CMV – and varicella – pneumonitis tend to be diffuse and bilateral and do not cavitate.

Answers – Case History 12 (5 marks)

1.
Best answer: **Bronchoscopy**
Accepted answers: Chest CT/Urinary hydroxy-indolic acid
Rejected answers: Ventilation perfusion scan/Liver ultrasound

2.
Best answers: **Bronchial carcinoid/Bronchial adenoma**
Accepted answers: Carcinoid/Benign endobronchial tumour
Rejected answer: Bronchial carcinoma

Bronchial carcinoid is a low-grade malignant tumour of the APUD system which may produce serotonin or ACTH. The other end of the spectrum represents a small cell carcinoma. These tumours are usually endobronchial and present with haemoptysis or localised obstruction. The serotonin secretion may produce local pulmonary fibrosis or endocardial/valve fibrosis of the left heart. Full-blown carcinoid syndrome is rare. The benign, Class I carcinoid is ten times commoner in females and the five-year survival rate is 95%. Therapy is by resection.

RESPIRATORY MEDICINE ANSWERS: DATA INTERPRETATIONS

Answers – Data Interpretation 1 (4 marks)

1. B Sleep apnoea
2. E Hypothyroidism

Sleep apnoea typically occurs in obese patients, more commonly in men. Hypoventilation and de-saturation occurs during REM sleep. Loud snoring and morning headaches are typical findings, daytime blood gases are normal. Underlying diseases such as neuromuscular disorders, hypothyroidism, (macrocytosis and hypercholesterolaemia) acromegaly, alcohol and sedative drugs need to be excluded.

Answers – Data Interpretation 2 (4 marks)

1.
Best answer: **Extra-pulmonary restrictive defect**
Accepted answer: Restrictive defect
Rejected answer: Obstructive defect

2.
Best answer: **Ankylosing spondylitis**
Accepted answer: Pleural encasement
Rejected answer: Pulmonary fibrosis

Reduced lung volumes with normal FEV_1/FVC coefficient indicate a restrictive defect. The normal transfer factors indicate that this is not due to parenchymal disease.
<u>Upper lobe lung disease:</u>
Progressive massive fibrosis (Silicosis)
Ankylosing spondylitis
Sarcoid
TB
Extrinsic allergic alveolitis (Chronic)
Mnemonic **PASTE**

Answers – Data Interpretation 3 (4 marks)

1. D Allergic broncho-pulmonary aspergillosis
2. A Sputum microscopy and culture

Differential diagnosis of a **pulmonary-renal syndrome** can be split into systemic diseases (i.e. Goodpasture's syndrome, vasculitides), primary pulmonary pathology (carcinoma, infection) which may cause secondary renal impairment or glomerulonephritis and primary renal pathology with secondary lung involvement (pulmonary oedema, embolism, metastasis).

ABPA is a hypersensitivity reaction to the fungus characterised by mucoid plugs and central bronchiectasis. It typically affects young asthmatic men.

Answer – Data Interpretation 4 (2 marks)

1. B Occupational asthma

The patient has evidence of mild airway obstruction at rest, with increased reactivity in the methacholine test. A hyperreactive system should have normal valves unless provoked.

Other differentials of a 'veterinarian' for MRCP include brucellosis, EAA, psittacosis, rabies and Orf.

Answers – Data Interpretation 5 (4 marks)

1.
Best answer: **High anion gap acidosis**
Accepted answers: Lactic acidosis/Partially compensated metabolic acidosis
Rejected answers: Mixed metabolic and respiratory acidosis

2.
Best answer: **Salicylate poisoning**
Accepted answer: Lactic acidosis
Rejected answer: Hypoglycaemia

In **salicylic acid poisoning** there is initially a respiratory alkalosis due to direct stimulation of the respiratory centre. Trying to compensate, the body reduces the bicarbonate buffer. In addition to the acidic effect of the salicylate itself, there is uncoupling of oxidative phosphorylation of carbohydrates. Increased fat metabolism results in high production of ketones which can no longer be neutralised and a profound metabolic acidosis ensues.
Anion gap: $[Na^{+}+K^{+}]-[Cl^{-}+HCO_3^{-}]$ = 40 mmol/l.

Answers – Data Interpretation 6 (4 marks)

1. D Bone marrow biopsy
2. B Chronic lymphocytic leukaemia

The diagnosis of **CLL** requires a lymphocytosis of > 10 x 10^9/l and > 30% lymphocytes in bone marrow. Presentation is usually insidious with lymphadenopathy and/or hepatosplenomegaly. It is a leukaemic form of a low-grade non-Hodgkin's lymphoma.

Answers – Data Interpretation 7 (4 marks)

1. D Re-breathing from paper bag
2. A Hyperventilation

The patient is hypocapnic without evidence of hypoxia or tachycardia. In the absence of these, the most likely cause is **hyperventilation**, with pulmonary embolus being the main differential diagnosis although this is less likely in the first trimester.

Answers – Data Interpretation 8 (5 marks)

1. C Mycoplasma pneumonia
2. A Direct Coombs' test

In **mycoplasma** infection, the presence of cold agglutinins results in haemolysis. This occurs *in vivo* with cooling of the blood in the periphery. Blood samples also frequently show haemolysis by the time they arrive in the lab. There is often a discrepancy between dramatic changes on the chest X-ray and relative well-being of the patient. Treatment is with macrolide antibiotics (erythromycin).

Answer – Data Interpretation 9 (4 marks)

1. E Subcutaneous salbutamol injections and anaesthetic assessment

The patient has a **severe asthma attack**. The 'normal' pCO_2 in a young patient with 'silent chest' indicates CO_2 retention and failure of the respiratory reserve. Urgent ventilation has to be considered.

Answers – Data Interpretation 10 (4 marks)

1.

Best answer: **Allergic broncho-pulmonary aspergillosis**
Accepted answers: Fungal infection/TB/Occupational asthma/Churg-Strauss syndrome
Rejected answers: Ankylosing spondylitis/Invasive aspergillosis, Aspergilloma

2.

Best answers: **Aspergillus precipitins/Prick test/Sputum microscopy/High-resolution CT**
Accepted answer: CT thorax
Rejected answers: Blood cultures/Tine test

ABPA is a hypersensitivity reaction to the ubiquitous fungus. Hyphae are present in the sputum, proximal bronchiectasis is a late complication. Occupational asthma and vasculitis are unlikely to produce sputum and should show some response to bronchodilators.

Answers – Data Interpretation 11 (4 marks)

1. A Emphysema
2. D α_1-antitrypsin deficiency

A young patient has increased lung volumes, reduced CO transfer coefficient and an obstructive pattern. The features are of **emphysema**. In a patient of this age, α_1-ATD has to be excluded.

Answer – Data Interpretation 12 (2 marks)

1. C Myasthenia gravis

The patient has alveolar hypoventilation. Associated with diplopia, this indicates a neuromuscular disorder. The likeliest is **myasthenia gravis**, possible differentials include botulism or overdose of muscle relaxants. Guillain-Barré syndrome would produce sensory signs and more extensive peripheral involvement before affecting the ocular muscles.

Answers – Data Interpretation 13 (5 marks)

1. C Relapsing polychondritis
2. A Normal appearances

An elderly patient with a systemic inflammatory disease has evidence of airways obstruction on forced expiration. However, resting lung volumes and gas transfer and saturation are normal. This indicates expiratory airways collapse. In combination with the systemic symptoms, this is highly suggestive of **relapsing polychondritis**. It can affect all cartilaginous structures, most commonly nose, ears and trachea. Biopsy shows a small vessel necrotizing vasculitis.

Episcleritis, arteriopathy and dilation of the cardiac valve rings also occur.

Answer – Data Interpretation 14 (3 marks)

1. E Arterial blood gases and iv erythromycin

Infection with ***Legionella pneumophila*** is characterised by signs of a chest infection (usually in smokers or patients with pre-existing lung disease) with systemic involvement. The classic MRCP-triad consists of hyponatraemia, abdominal pain and haematuria. Treatment is with macrolide antibiotics.

Answers – Data Interpretation 15 (4 marks)

1. B Pulmonary haemorrhage
2. D Hereditary haemorrhagic telangiectasia

HHT (Oslo-Weber-Rendu) is an autosomal dominant condition with telangiectatic changes mainly throughout the GI tract (lips!) but with associated pulmonary AV-malformation. The patients present with recurrent haemorrhage and iron deficiency anaemia. Increase in transfer coefficient (KCO) is seen in pulmonary haemorrhage, polycythaemia and increased blood flow through the lungs and asthma. KCO is the amount of CO taken up by the lungs (TCO) corrected for lung volume.

Answers – Data Interpretation 16 (4 marks)

1. C Arterial blood gases
2. D Pulmonary fibrosis

The patient presents sub-acutely after being started on **non-steroidal anti-inflammatory treatment**. Complications of this include precipitation of asthma, GI-bleed, deterioration of renal function, sodium & fluid retention and allergic reaction. ESR would be useful to confirm a flare-up of the disease, whereas the blood gases are unlikely to provide any further information in the context of normal pulse oximetry and pulmonary function tests. A single normal lung function measurement does not exclude bronchospasm, which may be intermittent.

Drugs that induce pulmonary fibrosis are nitrofurantoin and immune suppressants (bleomycin, cyclophosphamide and busulfan). This is a *long-term* complication.

Answers to Data Interpretation 17 (4 marks)

1. C D-dimer levels
2. B Pulmonary embolus

The patient is hypoxic with compensatory hyperventilation. The most likely diagnosis is **pulmonary embolus**. D-dimer levels are likely to be elevated and are the least invasive test. CT- angiogram is unlikely to pick up small emboli. If there remains clinical doubt the definitive investigation is a standard pulmonary angiogram.

Pregnancy is not an absolute contraindication to VQ-scanning, as the radiation dose to the fetus is low.

Answer – Data Interpretation 18 (3 marks)

1. D Drug side-effects

The prophylactic treatment for thromboses in anti-phospholipid syndrome is **aspirin**. This is confirmed by the prolonged bleeding time. The prolongation of APTT is a false positive result as the lupus anti-coagulant interferes with the test.

Causes for pulmonary eosinophilia include a number of drugs (commonest antibiotics and NSAIDs), fungal and parasite infection, vasculitis, rarely asthma and the benign, self-limiting idiopathic Loeffler syndrome.

Answers – Data Interpretation 19 (4 marks)

1. A Barium swallow
2. D Whipple's disease

The patient has a microcytic anaemia and dysphagia – the upper GI-tract needs to be assessed. Causes of basal lung fibrosis include all the connective tissue diseases; cryptogenic fibrosing alveolitis, asbestosis, drug-induced fibrosis and causes of **chronic aspiration**. Systemic sclerosis is less likely with a normal CRP and a microcytic anaemia. Tylosis is an autosomal dominant syndrome of hyperkeratosis of the palms and soles of the feet which is associated with carcinoma of the oesophagus.
Whipple's disease has associations with sacro-iliitis, sero-negative arthropathy, clubbing and erythema nodosum, but not pulmonary fibrosis.

Answers – Data Interpretation 20 (5 marks)

1. E O_2 administration
2. D iv doxapram

The patient has **Type II respiratory failure**. The main respiratory drive in this context is hypoxia. The commonest cause for removing the respiratory stimulant is administration of high concentrations of oxygen either directly or during nebulising of bronchodilators, which will cause acute worsening of the respiratory failure. Intravenous respiratory stimulants have to be admitted with close monitoring and great caution. Intubation in Type II failure is controversial and usually only recommended if there is an immediate correctable cause.

Answer – Data Interpretation 21 (2 marks)

1. E Histoplasmosis

Histoplasma capsulatum is endemic in North and South America and, to a lesser degree, in Africa and Australia. It is mainly found in bird and bat droppings ('bat-cave disease') and in soil. Infection may be asymptomatic, but commonly presents with an acute febrile pneumonia. In immune-compromised patients, dissemination may occur. Sputum microscopy is often unhelpful, but lung biopsy usually shows small yeast cells. The lung lesions calcify.

Answers – Data Interpretation 22 (5 marks)

1. B Carbon monoxide poisoning
2. B Exchange transfusion

CO-poisoning occurs acutely in attempted suicide (running car engine) or chronically with malfunctioning heating appliances. CO has a 250 times greater affinity to haemoglobin than O_2. Central cyanosis occurs with O_2 saturations of < 80% due to the dark colour of deoxy-haemoglobin. However, carboxyhaemoglobin has a cherry-red colour. The treatment of choice is hyperbaric oxygen, however in practice the availability is very limited. Removal of carboxyhaemoglobin in an emergency situation can be achieved by exchange transfusion.

Answers to Data Interpretation 23 (4 marks)

1. B Bronchoscopy and biopsy
2. B Alveolar cell carcinoma

Alveolar cell carcinoma accounts for 2–3% of lung tumours. Chest X-ray may show a solitary nodule, but a diffuse area of consolidation is common and these tumours can produce large amounts of mucoid secretion. The pneumonic form has a poor prognosis.

Answers – Data Interpretation 24 (4 marks)

1. C Extrinsic allergic alveolitis
2. A Apical fibrosis

EAA is a hypersensitivity reaction, usually to fungi (farmers, malt workers, cheese workers, the list is endless) or animal protein (pigeons). The *acute* form presents with fever and flu-like symptoms shortly after exposure to the allergen. *Chronic* exposure causes fibrosis of the upper aspects of the lungs. Causes of apical fibrosis include tuberculosis (calcification!), sarcoidosis (usually mid-zone), ankylosing spondylitis (often cavitating), EAA and other inhaled agents except for asbestos.
Mnemonic **PASTE: P**MF, **A**nkylosing **S**pondylitis, **S**arcoid, **T**B, **E**AA.

RHEUMATOLOGY ANSWERS: CASE HISTORIES

Answers – Case History 1 (10 marks)

1. D Blood cultures
2. D Traumatic tap
3. C Behçet's disease
4. B Systemic steroids
5. A Superior sagittal sinus thrombosis

Most venereal diseases cause *painless* genital ulcers. Gonorrhoea causes a purulent discharge. However a systemic infection must be excluded.

The important differentials of eosinophilia are allergy (drugs!), parasites (including fungi and malaria), vasculitis and Hodgkin's disease.

The combination of painful (oro-) genital ulcers, polyarthritis and iritis should alert to the diagnosis of **Behçet's disease**. Other features are erythema nodosum, pustular skin rashes and a variety of neurological syndromes (brain stem and cord lesions, aseptic meningitis and encephalitis).

Treatment is with steroids or immune-suppressants, vascular occlusion is an important complication.

The development of sterile pustules at puncture sites is called pathergy and, although not always seen, is very typical of Behçet's.

Answers – Case History 2 (7 marks)

1. B Creatinine kinase
2. E Polymyositis
3. B Barium enema

Polymyositis is a systemic disease of striated muscle characterised by perivascular lymphocytic infiltration. It causes a myopathy which may be painful and dysphagia and myocarditis. It is commoner in women (x 2) and is associated with HLA-B8 and HLA-DR3.

If associated with skin changes (i.e. vasculitic changes of hands and fingers) and the notorious peri-orbital rash and oedema (a heliotrope is a small purple flower), it is termed 'dermatomyositis'. The majority of cases are idiopathic, but 10% is associated with underlying malignancy (GI-tract, thyroid, breast, lymphoma). It is also found in mixed connective tissue diseases.

Painful proxal myopathy is characteristic and the diagnosis is made by EMG and/or muscle biopsy. Muscle enzymes (CK, AST, LDH) are markedly elevated. ANA are positive in 60%, anti-Jo1 positive in 30%.

Differentials are polymyalgia rheumatica (slight elevation of CK only), myasthenia gravis (marked eye signs) and familial myopathies. Therapy is with steroids and treatment of an underlying malignancy.

In this case, the presence of the microcytic anaemia and abnormal liver should alert to a possible underlying carcinoma of the colon.

Answers – Case History 3 (9 marks)

1. C Systemic lupus erythematodes
2. E Renal biopsy
3. A Avascular necrosis
4. B Nephrotic syndrome

A young woman with a multi-system disorder affecting the CNS (supra- and infra-tentorial), joints and kidneys. There is a significant occupational history, however the normal CRP is strongly against an infective cause which would also not explain her pancytopenia.

HIV has to be considered but would not readily explain the impaired renal function and heavy proteinuria.

Systemic lupus erythematodes typically has a discrepancy between a raised ESR and a normal CRP and also causes a falsely positive VDRL (the test incorporates cardiolipin as part of the antigen in the immune-assay).

The patient has cerebral lupus and renal impairment. The joints are frequently affected in the acute phase and avascular necrosis is a rare, but well described complication, in particular if the patient has been on long-term steroid therapy.

Renal involvement may be due to minimal change, proliferative or membranous GN, and often determines the outcome of the disease.

A lumbar puncture may show an increased amount of protein, this will by no means be diagnostic and the renal biopsy is going to be abnormal in the presence of hypertension and proteinuria.

Answers – Case History 4 (8 marks)

1. C Urinary protein and acetylcholine receptor antibodies
2. D Drug-induced myasthenia
3. C Stop penicillamine
4. A Rheumatoid lung

A woman with auto-immune disease (RA, thyrotoxicosis) develops diplopia and proximal weakness with fatiguability. She is on penicillamine and has evidence of recognised side-effects (thrombocytopenia, hypoproteinaemia with renal impairment). **Drug-induced myasthenia** is more likely than myasthenia gravis, although primary MG cannot be excluded on the basis of the findings given. Patients with HLA-BW35 and DR1 are said to have a higher incidence of drug-induced myasthenia, patients with HLA-DR3 generally show a higher side-effect rate with penicillamine.

Lung changes found in rheumatoid arthritis are pleural effusions, pulmonary nodules, basal fibrosis and infection secondary to immune-suppression.

Causes for **basal fibrosis** include CFA, asbestosis, connective tissue diseases and drug side-effects (bleomycin, cyclophosphamide, nitrofurantoin).

Answers – Case History 5 (6 marks)

1. B Small bowel biopsy
2. D Whipple's disease
3. A Tetracycline

Whipple's disease is caused by infection with *Tropheryema whippelii* which can be demonstrated on a PAS stain of a small bowel biopsy as pink material within macrophages. A related polyarthropy or spondylarthropy may precede the gastrointestinal symptoms. A polyserositis similar to FMF can be seen with fever, pleural and pericardial effusions, however presentation in FMF is usually at a young age whereas Whipple's disease classically manifests in men in the 4th and 5th decade. Malabsorption with diarrhoea and steatorrhoea is common.

Therapy is with protracted courses (three to six months) of oral antibiotics.

Answers – Case History 6 (6 marks)

1. E Churg-Strauss syndrome
2. D Anti-neutrophil-cytoplasmatic antibodies (ANCA)
3. A Degree of renal involvement

The patient has a multi-system disease with predominant renal involvement. The features are most consistent with a vasculitis, the presence of asthma-like symptoms and eosinophilia indicate **Churg-Strauss syndrome**. It is a granulomatous vasculitis affecting small to medium-sized vessels, clinical presentation is similar to PAN (= non-granulomatous). All organs can be affected, prognosis is determined by the progression of the renal failure, lung involvement is more common than with PAN.

Treatment is with steroids and immuno-suppressants.

Answers – Case History 7 (9 marks)

1.
Best answers: **ECG/ASO-titre**
Accepted answers: Echocardiogram/Blood cultures/Auto-antibody screen
Rejected answer: Joint aspirate

2.
Best answer: **Rheumatic fever**
Accepted answers: Post-streptococcal reactive arthritis/Chronic sepsis
Rejected answers: Still's disease/Infective endocarditis

3.
Best answer: **Chorea minor (Sydenham)**
Accepted answer: Brain abscess
Rejected answer: Meningitis

4.
Best answer: **Oral penicillin to the age of 20**
Accepted answer: Extended penicillin therapy
Rejected answer: Steroids

Rheumatic fever is a hypersensitivity reaction following two to three weeks after an infection with β-haemolysing group A streptococci. It affects heart (peri-, myo- or endocarditis), joints (polyarthritis), CNS (Chorea minor) and skin and subcutaneous tissues. A typical rash is erythema marginatum (pink annular rash over the trunk), but erythema nodosum can also be seen.

Prognosis is determined by the extent of endocardial involvement leading to valve defects (80% mitral, 20% aortic) which is a late manifestation. In the acute phase, an ECG is more important than an echocardiogram to demonstrate the prolonged PR interval, while valvular defects have not developed. Pericardial effusions, however, may be seen.

The diagnosis of rheumatic fever is made under combination of two major or one major and two minor of the Duckett-Jones criteria (American Heart Association) with evidence of a preceding streptococcal infection.

Major criteria	**Minor criteria**
1. Carditis	1. Fever
2. Polyarthritis	2. Arthralgia
3. Chorea minor	3. Raised ESR/CRP
4. Subcutaneous (Aschoff) nodules	4. Prolonged PR-interval
5. Erythema marginatum/annulare	5. Previous history of rheumatic fever

Haemolytic group A streptococci usually cause pharyngitis which, in the acute phase, can be demonstrated by throat swab, in the sub-acute phase a rising antibody titre is the examination of choice. Systemic infection causes scarlet fever.

RHEUMATOLOGY ANSWERS: DATA INTERPRETATIONS

Answers – Data Interpretation 1 (5 marks)

1. D Lyme disease
2. C Borrelia serology

First described in 1975 in **Lyme**, Connecticut, the disease is caused by *Borrelia burgdorferi* and transmitted by the Ixodes tic. If observed the rash, erythema chronicum migrans, is diagnostic. This may be followed by a variety of neurological symptoms as well as carditis and relapsing arthritis. Treatment should be performed early with penicillin or tetracycline.

Answers – Data Interpretation 2 (4 marks)

1. C Diffuse systemic sclerosis
2. D Blood pressure measurement

The distribution of autoantibodies is typical of **diffuse systemic sclerosis**. The limited cutaneous form (formerly CREST) typically shows antibodies against centromere. Raynaud's phenomenon and the skin stigmata are a prominent feature of the cutaneous form, but may be absent or preceded by systemic symptoms in the diffuse disease.

The main prognostic factor is currently lung involvement, the investigation of choice is a high-resolution CT. Monitoring of the blood pressure is mandatory as the patient may develop renal crisis.

The pulmonary fibrosis is typically in a basal distribution as with all the other connective tissue diseases.

Answers – Data Interpretation 3 (4 marks)

1. D Reactive amyloidosis
2. B Renal biopsy

Reactive (secondary) **amyloidosis** is found in conditions with chronic infection (i.e. bronchiectasis), chronic inflammation (i.e. inflammatory bowel disease) and some malignancies. Renal involvement leading to nephrotic syndrome or chronic renal failure and hepato-splenomegaly are typical, although in this patient the underlying lymphoma may be accountable for the latter.

Diagnosis is with biopsy showing the amorphous amyloid deposits which stain red with congo red and fluoresce green under polarised light.

Answers – Data Interpretation 4 (5 marks)

1. C Acute gout
2. D Joint aspiration and polarised light microscopy
3. B Diclofenac

The sudden onset of a monoarthritis on somebody who has been started on cytotoxic therapy for a condition with increased cell turnover is very suggestive of an **acute gout attack**. Chondrocalcinosis is a descriptive term which can be caused by a variety of different substances deposited in the cartilage. It occurs in the context of degenerative change, pseudogout, hyperparathyroidism, haemochromatosis and acromegaly, gout and Wilson's disease.

Gout crystals are negatively, calcium paraphosphate crystals positively bi-refringent. Treatment of acute gout is with non-steroidals.

Answers – Data Interpretation 5 (4 marks)

1. A Drug-induced lupus
2. C Alter current medication

Tuberose sclerosis has also been given the acronym EPILOIA as the syndrome is composed of **EPI**lepsy, **LO**w **I**ntelligence and **A**denoma sebaceum. The configuration of auto-antibodies indicates a drug-induced lupus, the likely offenders in this context are the anti-convulsants – phenytoin and carbamazepine.

Answers – Data Interpretation 6 (4 marks)

1. B Chest X-ray
2. D Loefgren syndrome

Loefgren syndrome (acute sarcoidosis) typically occurs in young women. The classic triad comprises of (ankle) arthritis, erythema nodosum and bi-hilar adenopathy. It is associated with pyrexia, cough and raised acute-phase proteins. A positive rheumatoid factor is present in approximately 15%, hyperuricaemia can also be seen in up to 25%.

ACE levels are useful for monitoring disease activity but as an unspecific mark of lung disease are not diagnostic for sarcoid.

Answers – Data Interpretation 7 (4 marks)

1. E Sjögren's syndrome
2. C Symptomatic therapy only

The positive auto-antibodies (> 1:80) indicate an autoimmune disease. The absence of double-stranded DNA antibodies is strongly against SLE. The normal hand X-ray does not rule out rheumatoid arthritis, but the presence of Ro & La antibodies suggest **primary Sjögren's syndrome**.

In the Schirmer test, strips of blotting paper are trapped with one end under the lower eyelids and a distance soaked with tears after five minutes is measured, normal is wetting of > 10 mm in five minutes, < 5 mm in five minutes is diagnostic of defective tear production.

Mikulicz syndrome is infiltration of salivary and tear ducts in lymphoma or CLL.

Heerfordt syndrome (uveo-parotid fever) is an extra-pulmonary manifestation of sarcoid with bilateral uveitis in the eyes, parotid gland infiltration which is occasionally associated with a lower facial nerve palsy.

Answers – Data Interpretation 8 (5 marks)

1.
Best answer: **Pauciarticular Still's disease**
Accepted answer: Still's disease
Rejected answers: Reiter's disease/Rheumatoid arthritis/Ankylosing spondylitis

2.
Best answer: **Urgent ophthalmology referral**
Accepted answers: Urgent rheumatology referral/Immune suppressant therapy
Rejected answers: Artificial tears/Systemic antibiotics

Pauciarticular **Still's disease** and adult Still's disease are often misdiagnosed for chronic sepsis due to the absence of rheumatological markers and the frequently present swinging pyrexia.

The systemic form seen in young children is associated with lymphadenopathy and splenomegaly and a characteristic macular erythema which is brought out by warmth and in the evening. In most forms, the joints are less swollen and painful than in rheumatoid arthritis. The chronic iritis seen in the pauciarticular form is a sight-threatening condition.

Answers – Data Interpretation 9 (4 marks)

1. D Haemochromatosis
2. B Liver biopsy

The patient presents with premature osteoarthrosis, mildly deranged liver function tests and diabetes mellitus. Iron overload in **haemochromatosis** is proven by estimating the dry iron content in the liver biopsy which will also detect associated serotic changes. Chronic hepatic porphyria = porphyria cutanea tarda, is the commonest of porphyrias and found in middle-aged men who drink too much. However, the diagnostic test is porphyrin levels in the urine although a liver biopsy will also be diagnostic. In acromegaly there is premature osteoarthrosis, however, due to cartilaginous overgrowth the joint spaces are characteristically widened.

Answers – Data Interpretation 10 (6 marks)

1. A Paget's disease
2. D Congestive cardiac failure
3. E Pelvic X-ray

An elderly gentleman presents with evidence of massively increased bone turnover, but a normal calcium and normal full blood count. This is associated with bone pain and increased osteoblastic activity in the pelvis. The features are of **Paget's disease of the bone**.

The biochemistry is not of osteomalacia. The borderline high PSA is perfectly consistent with prostatic hyperplasia. It does not exclude prostatic carcinoma, but there are no biochemical indicators of malignancy. A normal ESR essentially rules out myeloma.

The mildly raised liver function tests are in keeping with hepatic congestion due to the high-output cardiac failure which also explains the shortness of breath.

Answers – Data Interpretation 11 (4 marks)

1. E Takayasu's arteritis
2. C Arch-aortogram

A young woman with systemic inflammatory disease. This does not apply for coarctation, in the proximal form the blood pressure should be higher in the *right* arm anyway.

She is too young for polymyalgia or tertiary syphilis. Polymyositis does not affect the large vessels.

Takayasu's ('pulseless disease') is a granulomatous vasculitis affecting large vessels in young women. Arteriography will show wasting or occlusion of the aorta and its major branches.

Answers – Data Interpretation 12 (4 marks)

1. B Pseudoxanthoma elasticum
2. C Acute myocardial infarction

PXE is an inhomogeneous group of inherited disorders of elastic tissue. It affects skin, blood vessels, eyes and the heart. Although easily diagnosed by its lax skin which fails to recoil and a characteristic 'plucked chicken skin' appearance, the systemic complications are too often neglected. Intermittent claudication, angina and severe GI haemorrhages occur at an early age. Inheritance varies, but family screening and counselling is vital. Breaks in Bruch's membrane behind the retina causes *angioid streaks*, other causes include Marfan's, Ehler-Danlos disease and sickle-cell.

Answers – Data Interpretation 13 (4 marks)

1. E Osteomalacia
2. E Chest X-ray

The patient has features of alcoholic liver disease. In the context of hypocalcaemia, a proximal muscle weakness and bone pain is most likely due to **osteomalacia**. Loser zones are commonly seen in femoral necks, pubic rami, lower ribs and scapulae.

A raised ESR in a malnourished and immune-suppressed patient must alert to the possibility of active tuberculosis before other causes of infection are excluded.

Answers – Data Interpretation 14 (3 marks)

1. D Gonococcal arthritis
2. A Blood cultures

An acute monoarthritis in a young man, even without the pustular rash and the tenosynovitis is strongly suspicious for **gonococcal arthritis**. Other complications include epididymitis, meningitis, pelvic inflammatory disease and peri-hepatitis (Fitz-Hugh-Curtis syndrome).

Diagnosis is with urethral swabs and blood cultures, joint aspirates may be culture negative. Treatment is with penicillin, ciprofloxacin or tetracycline. Penicillin has the advantage of also covering syphilis, tetracycline also covers Chlamydia.

BIOCHEMICAL TESTS IN GENERAL MEDICINE

The following are only guidelines to the principle of each test. There is a great variation between hospitals, refer to your own lab before embarking on a physiological adventure. Several tests (i.e. insulin stress test and Tensilon test) are dangerous, particularly in the elderly and must only be performed with resuscitation facilities readily available. Many contraindications exist and these must be carefully excluded. Some tests are becoming obsolete in clinical practice.

Ammonium chloride acidification test — **Renal tubular acidosis I**

Principle: Oral administration of ammonium chloride results in a metabolic acidosis which is corrected by the kidneys and results in an acidic urine (pH < 5.4). In type I RTA the kidneys cannot excrete the acid load and the urine pH will fail to drop. Excretion is preserved in RTA type II

Criteria: Plasma bicarbonate must drop by at least 4mmol/l within 2 hours. Patient must not vomit during the test.

- Overnight fast, good hydration
- Baseline urine pH, if < 5.4 test not required
- 0.1 g/kg NH_4Cl is given orally
- Hourly urine pH-measurements for 8 hours

Positive if: urine pH does not fall < 5.4

Anion gap — **Metabolic acidosis**

Principle: Not actually a test as such, estimation of the anion gap is a useful way of estimating whether extra acidic substances (i.e. lactic acid, ketones, salicylates, methanol, ethylene glycol) are responsible for the acidosis.
<u>Normal:</u> 10–18 mmol/l, accounted for by phosphate and some organic acids

- $[Na^+ + K^+] - [HCO_3^- + Cl^-]$

<u>NB.</u> With a high anion gap the chloride is usually low (hypochloraemic acidosis). Chloride is not a standard test, as soon as it appears in the data, calculation of the anion gap is required!

Lactic acidosis type A: A for Anoxia
secondary to tissue hypoxia (shock, burns, hypoxia)
Lactic acidosis type B: B for Boisons
biguanides (metformin, phenformin)
= second cause for high anion gap in diabetics besides ketoacidosis, liver failure, poisoning (paracetamol, alcohol), lymphoma/leukaemia

Arginine infusion test **Growth hormone deficiency**

Principle: Intravenous administration of arginine stimulates the excretion of GH
Combined pituitary function test is usually preferred.

Dose: 30g arginine iv over 30 minutes

Positive if: GH-rise less than 15 mU/l

Breath Tests **Bacterial overgrowth/Malabsorption**

1. **Hydrogen breath test**

The only source of hydrogen in mammals is bacterial metabolism of carbohydrates in the gut. This normally occurs in the colon and up to 20% is absorbed into the blood and excreted via the lungs. In overgrowth of anaerobic bacteria in the small bowel an oral load of 75g of glucose (or 15g of lactulose) results in an early increase in hydrogen in the expired air as the sugar is already broken down before it reaches the colon.

2. **Radiocarbon breath test**

The patient is given 1g of xylose labelled with radioactive ^{14}C.
Normally xylose is absorbed to > 25% in small bowel, but not significantly metabolised.
In bacterial overgrowth the compound is broken down and radioactive $^{14}CO_2$ develops as a by-product, which again is excreted via the lungs.

Bromsulphthalein excretion test **Dubin-Johnson syndrome**

Principle: iv BSP is conjugated and excreted in the bile. Normally < 5% of injected dose present at 45 min. In any form of liver dysfunction this level remains high, in Dubin-Johnson syndrome it is said that after an initial drop the serum levels at 120 min. are higher than at 45 min. The test is risky and probably obsolete.

Captopril Test **Hyperaldosteronism**

Principle: Renin (an enzyme produced in the juxtaglomerular apparatus) cleaves angiotensinogen to angiotensin 1 which is converted in the lungs to angiotensin 2 by A-1 converting enzyme (ACE). A-2 is not only the most potent (known) vasoconstrictor, but also stimulates the secretion of aldosterone in the adrenals. Blockade of ACE results in a drop of aldosterone in healthy individuals and secondary (RAS and idiopathic) hyperaldosteronism.

In primary hyperaldosteronism (Conn's syndrome) the aldosterone levels are unaffected and baseline renin is low.

In renal artery stenosis (RAS) there is an exaggerated increase in renin following ACE-inhibition, as the compromised kidney is being starved even further of its compromised blood supply.

Criteria: Baseline aldosterone should be raised (>400 pmol/l)

- After bed-rest from at least midnight 08.00 am blood sample for baseline renin and aldosterone is taken in *supine* position
- 25 mg captopril orally
- After 120 min (*supine*) take further sample for renin and aldosterone

Normal: Aldosterone level below 400 pmol/l with further drop after captopril

Conn's: Aldosterone > 400 pmol/l, no drop after ACE inhibition

RAS: Aldosterone high, drops after captopril.

Renin doubles (or more) after captopril. In essential hypertension and increase of up to 150% of baseline may be seen.

Combined pituitary function test **Hypopituitarism**

Principle: Combination of

- insulin stress test for GH and cortisol
- TRH test for thyroid axis
- GN-RH test for gonadotrophic axis

Criteria: Evidence of hypopituitarism rather than end-organ failure.

Hypoglycaemia of < 2.2 mmol/l must be achieved, ideally with patient being symptomatic (iv glucose must be immediately available, if this needs to be

given continue the test, as hypoglycaemic stress was adequate to induce hormone release).
Many contraindications (see *insulin stress test*).

- iv cannula sited at least 30 min prior to test to reduce stress of blood sampling
- After 30 min. baseline samples for GH and cortisol, TSH, LH and FSH and glucose
- Start test with injection of 0.15 U/kg soluble insulin i.v., 200 μg TRH and 100 μg GN-RH
- Repeat blood samples from cannula at 30, 60, 90 and 120 min.

Positive if:
1. GH rise < 15mU/l / GH peak < 20 mU/l
2. Cortisol rise < 200 nmol/l (basal level should double)/Cortisol peak < 550 nmol/l
3. TSH response
   exaggerated (1° hypothyroidism)
   reduced (2° hypothyroidism)
   delayed (3° hypothyroidism)
   absent (hyperthyroidism)
   → see *TRH test* for details
   Gonadotrophin response (see *GN-RH test)*

Corticotrophin releasing hormone test **Cushing's disease vs. syndrome**

Principle: Intravenous CRH stimulates the secretion of ACTH by the anterior pituitary resulting in an increase in cortisol.
A pituitary adenoma will respond by releasing an overshoot of ACTH resulting in a marked increase in serum cortisol = **Cushing's disease**, pituitary driven adrenal hyperplasia
An autonomous adrenal adenoma or ectopic ACTH secretion will not be influenced by additional ACTH = **Cushing's syndrome**

Dexamethasone suppression test **Cushing's disease vs. syndrome**

Principle: Dexamethasone, a potent synthetic steroid should suppress ACTH secretion resulting in a drop in serum cortisol. The feedback mechanism is impaired in pituitary driven hypercortisolism (Cushing's disease) and absent in adrenal adenoma and ectopic ACTH production.

Criteria: Basal serum cortisol must be high to begin with, otherwise a high ACTH is secondary to adrenal failure
All cortisol samples should be taken between 8.00 and 9.00 a.m.

- The cortisol levels in a normal person should drop by more than 50%.

a. low dose dexamethasone test
Dose: 2 mg/day orally for 48 hours (either single dose at night or 0.5 mg qds)
Positive if: Serum cortisol fails to suppress below 50% of baseline / below 125 nmol/l

NB: this does not differentiate between a pituitary or adrenal/ectopic cause

b. high dose dexamethasone test
Criteria: Abnormal low dose dexamethasone test
Often this follows immediately on from the low-dose test on day three
Dose: 8 mg/day orally for 48 hours (either single dose at night or 2 mg qds)
Positive if: serum cortisol fails to suppress below 50% of baseline / below 125 nmol/l
→ this is in favour of adrenal/ectopic production, as most (2/3) of pituitary adenomas suppress on the high dose test

Dicopac® -Test **Pernicious anaemia**
Principle: The body is saturated with an im injection of vitamin B_{12}. A mixture of ^{58}Co-labelled B_{12} and a compound of ^{57}Co labelled B_{12}/intrinsic factor is given orally. In pernicious anaemia there will be differential excretion of the two isotopes in the urine (i.e. the former will be abnormally low). In other causes of B_{12} deficiency (i.e. terminal ileal disease, bacterial overgrowth) urinary excretions of both substances will be low. For full details see *Schilling-test.*
Positive if: Excreted dose of radioactive B_{12} < 8% (24hr urine collection)

Ellsworth-Howard test **Pseudo-/Hypoparathyroidism**

PTM increases urine phosphate excretion. This is mediated via the intracellular second messenger cyclic-AMP, which also appears in the urine.

Normal excretion: urinary PO_4^{3-} 13–42 nmol/day, urinary c-AMP 0.5 nmol/mmol creatinine

Principle: Hypoparathyroidism (reduced/absent endogenous parathormone): The infusion of parathormone results in a 10–20 fold increased urinary excretion of PO_4^{3-} and c-AMP.

Pseudohypoparathyroidism (end-organ resistance): endogenous parathormone is present, but ineffective. Administration of exogenous PTH makes no difference → no increased PO_4^{3-} excretion in the urine. Two types:

- Type 1: receptor defect results in complete failure of target cell response
  → no c-AMP is produced in the cell, no urinary increase of c-AMP or PO_4^{3-}
- Type 2: receptor intact, but c-AMP ineffective
  → rise in urinary c-AMP, urinary PO_4^{3-} unaltered

Faecal fat excretion **Steatorrhoea**

Principle: Normal daily fat excretion is less than 7 g/day. Steatorrhoea can be due to maldigestion (pancreas) or malabsorption (small bowel). The reliability of the test is impaired by daily variation of diet and difficulties collecting all the samples. Usually an average over 5 consecutive days is obtained.

Criteria: Normal diet containing 50-100 g fat/day (no more!) for at least three days prior to test.

Positive if: Total faecal fat > 10 g/d (> 30 g in 3 days)

Glucose suppression test **Acromegaly**

Principle: Growth hormone (GH) levels should drop in response to an increasing blood sugar. (See also OGTT)

- Overnight fast
- iv cannula sited at least 30 min. prior to test to reduce stress of blood sampling

- Basal glucose and GH-levels are taken
- 75g of glucose or equivalent carbohydrates are given orally in 250–300ml of fluid within five minutes
- Further glucose and GH levels at 30, 60, 90 and 120 minutes

Positive if: GH fails to suppress below 4 mU/l
False positive: severe hepatic or renal failure, drug addicts, levodopa therapy

Gonadotrophin releasing hormone (GN-RH) test **Amenorrhoea**

Principle: GN-RH should result in release of LH and FSH from the pituitary. Normal values vary greatly throughout the female cycle and between hospitals and normal ranges are usually given in the exam. Both values should roughly rise by more than 5 U/l into double figures. In primary ovarian failure basal gonadotrophins will be high, in pituitary failure there will be no response to GN-RH, in hypothalamic dysfunction there will be a normal or delayed response analogue to the TRH test.
Criteria: Low gonadotrophin levels, otherwise primary ovarian failure is present.

- Basal levels
- 100 μg GN-RH
- FSH and LH levels at 30, 60, 90 and 120 min.

Hypothalamic dysfunction: normal response
Pituitary failure/anorexia: absent/reduced response

Ham's test **Parox. nocturnal haemoglobinuria**

Principle: Acquired sensitivity of red cells to activated complement results in intravascular haemolysis. Haemolysis occurs during sleep (reduced oxygen tension) with dark urine in the morning. *In vitro* this manifests as a reduced tolerance to acidic media resulting in haemolysis at higher pH (less acidic) than normal erythrocytes.

Insulin stress test **Growth hormone (GH) deficiency**

Principle: Hypoglycaemia causes a physiological increase in the 'diabetogenic' hormones GH and cortisol. Usually performed as part of the *combined pituitary stimulation test.* Contraindicated in ischaemic heart disease, epilepsy and the frail and elderly!

- iv cannula sited at least 30 min. prior to test to reduce stress of blood sampling
- Baseline GH and glucose
- 0.15 U/kg soluble insulin iv
- Repeat samples at 30, 60, 90 120 min.

Criteria: Blood glucose < 2.2 mmol/l, ideally patient should be symptomatic (iv Glucose must be drawn up & ready, if it needs to be given, *continue sampling!*) If poor response, test can be repeated with 0.3 U/kg

Positive if: GH increases by less than 15 mU/l/peak value < 20 mU/l

Lactose tolerance test **Lactose intolerance**

Principle: The disaccharide lactose is split by lactase into galactose and glucose which is absorbed in the small bowel.

- Basal blood glucose
- 50 g of oral lactose
- Blood glucose should rise more than 1 mmol/l

Lumbar Puncture

	Normal	**Bacterial**	**Viral**
Colour	clear	pus	clear/turbid
Pressure	10–16 cm H_2O	↔/↑	↔
Protein	0.2–0.4 g/l	0.5–5 g/l	0.4–1 g/l
Glucose	> 60% of blood	< 40%	normal
Red cells	none	no	no
Lymphocytes	< 5/µl	<50/µl	10–100/µl
Polymorphs	none	300–3000/µl	occasional

	TB	SAH	traumatic tap
Colour	turbid, sticky	Xanthochromia after 4 hrs	blood
Pressure	↑	↔/↑	↔
Protein	0.5–3 g/l	0.2–0.5 g/l	0.2–0.5 g/l
Glucose	< 40%	normal	↔/↑
Red cells	no	yes	yes
Lymphocytes	100–300/μl	occasional	occasional
Polymorphs	0–200/μl	occasional	occasional

Nicotinic acid test **Gilbert's syndrome**

Principle: Unconjugated bilirubin levels rise (5–10 μmol/l) after administration of nicotinic acid to a peak (average 15–20 μmol/l) at *90 min* in normal persons. In Gilbert's the peak is higher (45–50 μmol/l) and occurs at *2–3 hours*.
Baseline is usually 20–25 μmol/l
A 1.5–2 fold increase is also seen on fasting (< 400 kcal/d for 3 days), normal levels < 25 μmol/l.

- 50 mg nicotinic acid iv
- Bloods at 60, 90, 120 and 360 min

Oral glucose tolerance test (OGTT) **Diabetes mellitus**

Random plasma glucose > 11mmol/l or fasting plasma glucose > 8 mmol/l
DM present, **OGTT not required**
Random plasma glucose < 8 mmol/l or fasting plasma glucose < 6 mmol/l
DM excluded, **OGTT not required**

Principle: Oral glucose load leads to an abnormal increase in plasma glucose levels in DM.
A mixture of glucose and its oligosaccharides is preferred to pure glucose as this is less osmolar, the patient is less likely to vomit and absorption is more reliable

- Patient on normal diet, overnight fast
- Basal plasma levels are taken

- 75g of glucose or equivalent carbohydrates are given orally in 250–300ml of fluid within five minutes, patient should sit or walk, if patient must lie down this should be on the right side in order to allow gastric emptying
- Further glucose levels at 30, 60, 90 and 120 minutes

Results:

Impaired glucose tolerance:	2 hr glucose > 8mmol/l, but <11mmol/l (normal fasting levels)
Diabetes mellitus:	2 hr glucose > 11mmol/l
'Lag storage curve':	Peak plasma glucose reached early (can be > 11mmol/l) 2 h glucose normal/lower than baseline often delayed hypoglycaemia (→ late samples required) Seen in: 'dumping syndrome' following gastric surgery, liver disease, some normals
Flat response:	Levels do not rise above 7mmol/l Seen in: patient lying on the left during test, vomiting, malabsorption, pituitary/adrenal failure

Osmolality (plasma) **Fluid overload/SIADH**

Principle: Useful normal value, particularly in combination with urine osmolality (see water deprivation test) The sum of the major electrolytes (for ease of calculation the cations are added and doubled to account for the corresponding anions) is added to the two major organic molecules.

Normal: 280–295 mosm/kg

- $[Na^+ + K^+] \times 2 + [Urea] + [Glucose]$

Osmotic resistance/fragility **Hereditary spherocytosis**

Principle: Due to an inherited membrane protein defect the cells 'swell' from a saucer to a spherical shape, thus reducing their cross-section (→ microcytosis). When introduced into an increasingly hypotonic medium the already 'swollen' cells tolerate the further influx of water less than normal cells and lyse earlier. This corrects with the addition of glucose.

Pentagastrin test **Abnormal gastric acid output**

Principle: Pentagastrin stimulates gastric secretion analogue to gastrin. In Zollinger-Ellison syndrome there is an overshoot 'peak acid output' (PAO), pernicious anaemia shows a reduced response.

- NG tube sited, collection of gastric secretions over 1 hour (basal acid output, BAO: < 5 mmol/h))
- 6 µg/kg pentagastrin s.c.
- gastric aspiration at 15, 30, 45 and 60 min.

Positive if: PAO > 60 mmol/h → Z-E syndrome
(also BAO > 15 mmol/h)
PAO < 10 mmol/h → pernicious anaemia, H_2-blockers, vagotomy, hypothyroidism

Peak acid output is defined as the two subsequent aspirates with the highest values.

Schilling Test **Vitamin B_{12} deficiency**

Principle: Dietary B_{12} is absorbed in the terminal ileum in the presence of intrinsic factor produced in the gastric mucosa.

1st part: After saturation of the body stores by an im injection of 1mg normal B_{12} a dose of radioactive ^{58}Co-labelled B_{12} is given orally. As the body is saturated by the injection, more than 10% of the radioactive dose should be excreted in the following 24hr urine collection

2nd part: If this is not the case the test is repeated with the addition of intrinsic factor. If excretion normalises, pernicious anaemia is confirmed.
If excretion still low, then there is either terminal ileal disease or overgrowth of bacteria metabolising the B_{12}. The latter is confirmed by repeating the test after oral antibiotics or by hydrogen breath test or small bowel aspiration for culture.

Both parts can be performed at the same time with a mixture ^{58}Co-labelled B_{12} and a compound of intrinsic factor and B_{12} which is labelled with ^{57}Co (Dicopac®-Test). In pernicious anaemia there will be differential excretion of the two isotopes, in other pathology both urinary excretions will be low.

Positive if: Excreted dose of radioactive B_{12} < 8% (24hr urine collection)

Secretin suppression test **Zollinger-Ellison syndrome**

Principle: Gastrin levels are normally suppressed by secretin. In Z-E there a paradoxical rise of greater than 100% occurs after injection of secretin.

Steroid suppression test **Hypercalcaemia**

Principle: Hypercalcaemia due to **sarcoidosis**, myeloma, hypervitaminosis D and Addison's disease (rare manifestation) suppress with high doses of steroids. Ectopic PTH suppresses to a lesser extent. Hyperparathyroidism (primary or tertiary) is unaffected. Metastatic bone involvement suppresses in 50%.

- Hydrocortisone 40 mg tds for ten days

Positive if: Ca^{2+} levels suppress to normal levels (< 2.55 mmol/l). The clinical context decides between sarcoid, vitamin D effects or myeloma.

Synacthen® test **Hypoadrenalism/Addison's disease**

Principle: Synthetic ACTH stimulates the adrenals and results in increased serum cortisol.
Failure of cortisol to rise in the short test can be due to primary adrenal failure (Addison's disease), adrenal suppression (i.e. steroid therapy) or long-standing hypopituitarism. The latter two are excluded by prolonged adrenal stimulation with the long test.

Criteria: Low serum cortisol

a. short Synacthen® test:

- Basal cortisol levels
- 250 µg tetracosactrin i.m.
- Cortisol levels at 30 and 60 min.

Positive if: Cortisol < 550nmol/l at 30 min, < 650 nmol/l at 60 min
If the test positive proceed to

b. long Synacthen® test

- Following short test 1 mg tetracosactrin depot is given i.m.
- Cortisol levels after further 24hr

Delayed response: hypopituitarism or exogenous steroids; no response: Addison's disease.

Tensilon® test **Myasthenia gravis**

Principle: Injection of a cholinesterase inhibitor increases the concentration of acetylcholine at the motor endplate by inhibition of its breakdown. Increase in muscle power (i.e. resolution of bilateral ptosis on upward gaze) occurs within seconds lasting several minutes. This type of drug is used in Anaesthetics as a depolarising muscle relaxant, it can cause severe bronchospasm or syncope and resuscitation facilities must be at hand.

- Edrophonium test dose 1 mg iv
- Edrophonium 10 mg iv bolus
- As the test is subjective, several observers should be present, control injection with saline can be performed if in doubt

TRH-test (Thyrotropin releasing hormone) **Hypothyroidism**

Principle: Assessment of hypothalamic-pituitary-thyroid axis After TRH the normal TSH should peak at 20 min (5–20 mU/l, increase > 2 mU/l over baseline) and drop steadily (60 min. value no lower than 1/3rd of 20 min peak).

- Basal TSH levels
- 200 µg TRH iv
- TSH levels after 20 and 60 min.

Results:

1° hypothyroidism:
basal TSH high, exaggerated and prolonged response to TRH

2° hypothyroidism (pituitary failure):
low baseline, minimal increase at 20 min (< 2 mU/l), back to baseline at 60 min.

3° hypothyroidism (hypothalamic dysfunction):
delayed rise in TSH with low 20 min and high 60 min value

hyperthyroidism:
flat response, no increase in TSH

Water deprivation test **Diabetes insipidus**

Principle: Test for investigation of polyuria/suspected defect in urinary concentration.
Restriction of water intake stimulates ADH-secretion resulting in increasing urine osmolality but maintained serum osmolality.

In **diabetes insipidus** ADH is absent (central form) or ineffective (nephrogenic form) and the kidneys fail to retain water. If the baseline plasma osmolality is low, DI is excluded. On fluid deprivation the plasma osmolality rises > 300 mosm/kg while the urine fails to concentrate.

If there is evidence of DI the administration of synthetic ADH (DDAVP, Vasopressin) will correct the defect in the central form, but will make no difference in the peripheral form as there is a receptor defect in the kidney.

Psychogenic polydipsia is easily distinguished as the plasma osmolality is low to begin with and will not rise above normal values. DDAVP is not required. Frequently the concentration gradient has been washed out of the kidney and prolonged fluid restriction is required. The patient may also secretly continue drinking during the test.

- Overnight fast
- Baseline weight and urine and plasma samples → if urine > 800 mosm/kg the kidneys can concentrate normally and the test can be stopped
- No food or water for 8 hours, 2-hourly measurements
- The test is stopped, if the urine > 800 mosm/kg or the patient has lost 5% of their body weight
- If urinary concentration does not occur in the presence of haemoconcentration 4μg DDAVP are given im

Results after 8hr fluid deprivation:

	Normal	Central D.I.	Nephrogenic D.I.	Polydipsia
Serum	280–295	305–320	305–320	270–295
Urine	800–1500	100–300	100–300	200–700
Urine after DDAVP	–	increased by > 10%	Unchanged as ineffective	–

Xylose absorption test **Malabsorption**

Principle:	D-xylose is rapidly absorbed and largely excreted in the urine. A 5g dose is usually preferred to 25 g as less osmotic side-effects. It is an unspecific and not very sensitive test for small bowel absorption
Normal:	> 25 % of oral dose excreted within five hours (> 12 % after two hours)

- Empty bladder
- 5 g (25 g) D-xylose in 200 ml water
- Urine collection of first two and further three hours

Two questions solve the dreaded family tree:

1. Are all generations affected (dominant)?
2. Is there male-to-male (father-to-son) transmission (autosomal)?

Autosomal Dominant Inheritance

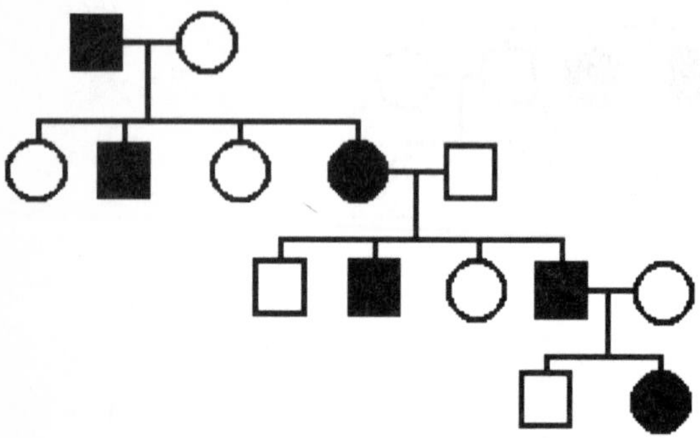

Key Features

- Both sexes are equally affected
- All generations are affected
- Children of an affected parent will have a 1:2 chance of developing the disease
- The transmission stops with an unaffected person

Examples:

Acute intermittent porphyria
Adult polycystic kidney disease
α1-Antitrypsin deficiency
C_1-esterase deficiency
Familial intestinal polyposis/Peutz-Jeghers syndrome
Hereditary spherocytosis
Hereditary telangiectasia
Huntingdon's chorea
Marfan's syndrome/Osteogenesis imperfecta tarda
Medullary carcinoma thyroid/Multiple endocrine neoplasia
Neurofibromatosis/Tuberose sclerosis/von-Hippel Lindau (Sturge-Weber sporadic)
Rotor's disease
von Willebrand's disease

Autosomal Recessive Inheritance

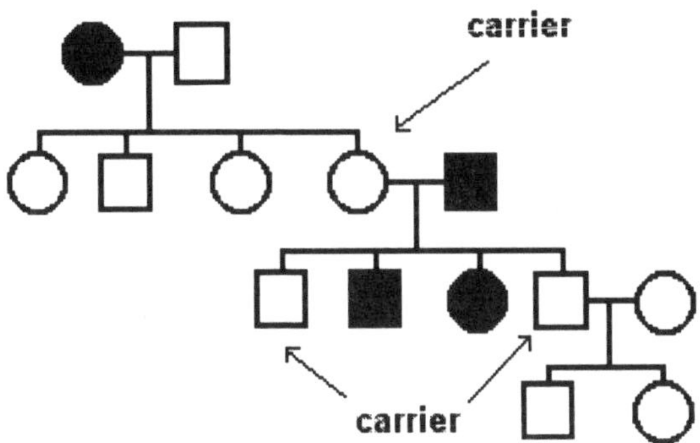

Key Features:

- Both sexes are equally affected
- NOT every generation is affected
- Unaffected persons can transmit the abnormal gene = heterozygous carriers
- One parent carrier: 1:4 (25%) of children carriers
- One affected parent (homozygous): All children carriers
- Both parents carriers: 1:2 (50%) of children carriers
  1:4 (25%) of children affected,
  1:4 (25%) of normal genes
- One affected parent, one carrier: 1:2 (50%) of children carriers
  1:2 (50%) of children affected

Examples:

Congenital adrenal hyperplasia
Cystic fibrosis
Dubin-Johnson syndrome/Gilbert's syndrome
Haemochromatosis/Wilson's disease
Hurler's disease
Infantile polycystic disease
Sickle cell disease/β-thalassaemia

Most metabolic disorders:

Fructose intolerance
Phenylketonuria, cystinuria
Glycogen storage diseases
Lysosomal storage diseases (Gaucher's, Niemann-Pick, Tay-Sachs) except Fabry's disease (X-recessive)

X-linked recessive Inheritance

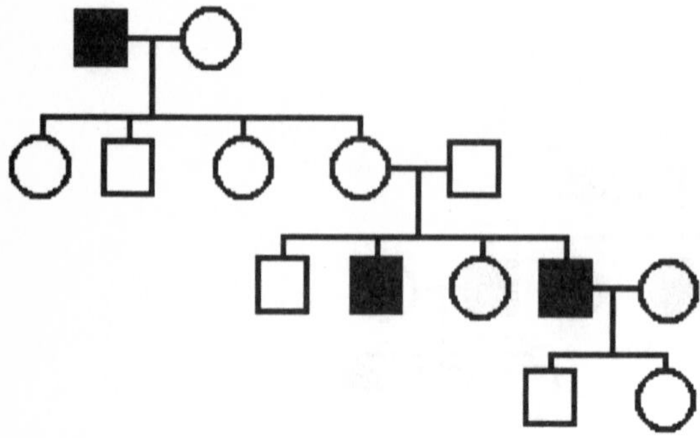

Key Features:

- Usually one generation skipped = Knight's move pattern
- No male-to-male transmission
- Virtually only males affected, females usually carriers only
- Maternal carrier:
  1:2 sons affected, the others healthy (no male carriers)
  1:2 daughters will be carriers
- Affected father
  all sons healthy (no male-to-male transmission)
  all daughters carriers (!)
- A woman can only be affected (= homozygous), if her father is affected AND her mother carries at least one abnormal gene (usually consanguinity)

Examples:

Becker's/Duchenne's muscular dystrophy
Fabry's disease
G6P-dehydrogenase deficiency
Haemophilia A & B
Hunter's disease
Idiopathic sideroblastic anaemia
Lesch-Nyhan syndrome
Nephrogenic diabetes insipidus
Red-green colour blindness

X-linked dominant Inheritance

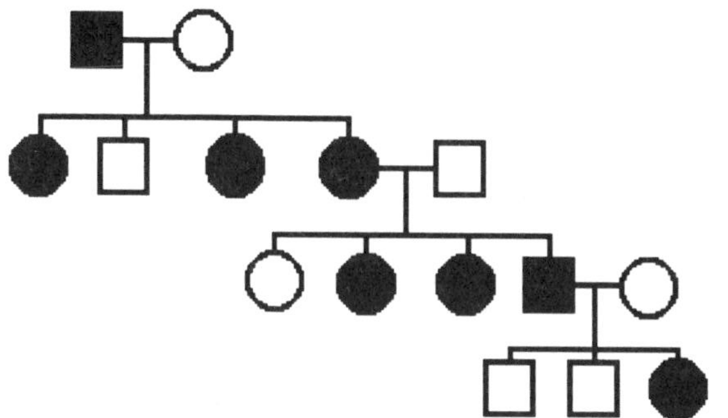

Key Features:

- All generations affected, if daughters present
- No male-to-male transmission
- Most cases will be females

- Affected father
  all sons healthy
  all daughters affected

- Affected mother:
  1:2 children affected if heterozygous
  all children affected if homozygous

Examples:
Chronic granulomatous disease
Pseudohypoparathyroidism
Vitamin D resistant rickets

HISTOLOGICAL STAINS

Technique	Application
Cresyl blue (supravital stain)	Reticulocytes: blue reticulation Heinz bodies: blue (splenectomy, G-6 PDH def., toxic/met-Hb)
Congo red	Amyloid: red (apple-green under polarised light → positive birefringent)
Gram	Gram-positive cocci: blue (staphylococci = grapes, streptococci = chains, pneumococci = buns) Gram-negative cocci: red (diplococci: Neisseria meningitidis and gonorrhoeae)
Grimelius	APUD-cell tumours (carcinoid, islet cell tumours)
Grocott	See silver
Indian ink	Fungi: pale on black background
Massou-Fontana-Silver	Melanin: black (melanoma)
Periodic acid Schiff (PAS)	*Tropheryma whippelii* (Whipple's disease): pink bodies within macrophages Fungi: red
Pearl's stain (= Prussian blue)	Iron: dark blue Liver: Haemochromatosis and other causes of iron overload Ring sideroblasts (hereditary, myeloproliferation, toxic/drugs, CTD) Pappenheimer bodies in erythrocytes post-splenectomy

Rose bengal	Mucus: pink (sicca syndrome and Sjögren's)
Romanowsky	Basophilic stippling: dark blue dots in erythrocytes (lead poisoning) Howell-Jolly bodies: blue nuclear fragments (hyposplenism) also a standard bone marrow stain Multiple myeloma: binucleate cells with large amount of blue cytoplasm = 'owl's eyes' appearance (> 8% diagnostic)
Rubeonic acid	Copper: brown (Wilson's disease)
Silver stain	Fungi (incl. histoplasmosis)/ yeasts: brown/black, linear Pneumocystis: black, oval
Modified Ziehl-Neelson (Z-N)	Acid fast bacilli (= stain is acid fast, not bacilli; TB, leprosy) cryptosporidium

REFERENCES

1. Whitby L.G., Percy-Robb I.W., Smith A.F. *Lecture notes on clinical chemistry.* 3rd ed. Blackwell scientific publications, Oxford.
2. Zilva J.F., Pannall P.R., Mayne P.D. *Clinical chemistry in diagnosis and treatment.* 5th ed. Edward Arnold, London.
3. Thomas L. *Labor und Diagnose.* 5th ed. TH-Books Verlags-Gesellschaft, Frankfurt
4. Kumar P., Clark M. *Clinical Medicine.* 2nd ed. Bailliere Tindall, London.
5. Herold G. *Innere Medizin.* 1994, Gerd Herold, Köln.
6. Thomson A.D., Cotton R.E. *Lecture notes on pathology.* 3rd ed. Blackwell scientific publications, Oxford.
7. Govan A.D., MacFarlane P.S., Callander R. *Pathology illustrated.* 1st ed. Churchill Livingstone, Edinburgh.
8. Sandritter W., Thomas C. *Histopathologie.* 9th ed. Schattauer, Stuttgart.
9. Oxford textbook of medicine on CD-ROM. Version 1.1, Oxford University Press and Electric Publishing.
10. Firkin, B.G., Whitworth J.A. *Dictionary of Medical Eponyms,* 1st ed. Glaxo/Parthenon, Carnforth.

INDEX

Numbers given are for pages on which relevant question or answer appear. The word shown may not always be used in the question, but may appear in the explanatory answer. Numbers in bold type are for Major References within the text.